TRADITIONAL CHINESE HAND AND FOOT MASSAGE

by Wu Gengwei
Hao Dongfang

FOREIGN LANGUAGES PRESS   BEIJING

First Edition 2001
Translated by Wang Tai

Home Page:
http://www.flp.com.cn
E-mail Addresses:
Info@flp.com.cn
Sales@flp.com.cn

ISBN 7-119-01945-7
©Foreign Languages Press, Beijing, 2001
Published by Foreign Languages Press
24 Baiwanzhuang Road, Beijing 100037, China
Distributed by China International Book Trading Corporation
35 Chegongzhuang Xilu, Beijing 100044, China
Printed in the People's Republic of China

ABOUT THE AUTHORS

Wu Gengwei was born in Beijing in 1966 and began learning traditional Chinese medicine from his grandfather Zhang Ding-wen when he was 12 years old. He received his medical education at the Beijing University of Traditional Chinese Medicine where he received a medical bachelor's degree. Mr. Wu is presently a postgraduate student of pedagogy at Ziho University in Japan. He is a member of the Japanese Research Society of Physical and Mental Anxiety, the Japanese Society of Human Body Sciences, the Japanese Society of Sport Psychology, and the Japanese Society of Medical Qigong.

Hao Dongfang, born in Beijing in 1966, is a physician for the Chinese National Swimming Team. He graduated from the Beijing University of Traditional Chinese Medicine with a bachelor's degree in 1989.

CONTENTS

FOREWORD

Through development and improvement over thousands of years, traditional Chinese medicine gradually divided into many branches. Hand and foot massage is a comparatively young member of this ancient healing art. Because of the simplicity and practicality of this therapy, it has long been very wide spread among the ordinary people of China, although it was not admitted to the honored ranks of the classical tradition of medicine due to certain historical reasons.

In 1987, we were fascinated by this therapy as soon as we watched a demonstration of it for the first time. Without even questioning the patients about their symptoms, the practitioner could make accurate diagnoses of their ailments simply by observing the abnormal changes of color and shape of their hand and feet. What impressed us even more was the fact that the patients' sufferings could be quickly relieved merely by applying this special massage therapy to their hands and feet.

With a deep interest in exploring the treasure store of traditional Chinese medicine and developing our national culture, we embarked on systematic study and compilation of traditional hand and foot massage therapy.

The imformation and materials gathered in this volume were mainly collected from folk medicine sources. Although the techniques were useful in practice, the information on them was disorganized and scattered. Sometimes, it was difficult to interpret. At the same time, the information and materials included in the classic sources of Chinese medical literature were fragmentary, superficial and often incoherent.

Throughout the course of our work, we used the basic theories of traditional Chinese medicine as the theoretical guide times, reinforced by extensive clinical practice as the objective standard with which to repeatedly compare and authenticate the unsophisticated lore of the common people, to screen and preserve the sound scientific knowledge and effective therapeutic measures of this folk tradition, and to discard the unscientific and useless components.

We first summarized the diagnostic methods and grouped them under the headings of inspection, palpation, pressing and motion tests. We also explained the therapeutic mechanism of hand and foot massage from the scientific angle to show its scientific nature and to explain it as an objective approach to healing which has long been well understood by the common people. At the same time, we utilized modern theories and techniques to enrich and develop this ancient therapy, including biological holographic methods of diagnosis and treatment, and reflective therapy involving the soles of the feet. As a result, a complete and independent branch of traditional Chinese medicine with a specific and distinctive nature, has emerged.

Movement and development are basic to the natures of all substances in the world, and the continued existence of any substance is always dependent on getting rid of the stale and taking in the fresh so that it may develop and maintain exuberant vitality.

In the spirit of gratitude to the researchers who came before us, we diligently studied and developed traditional hand and foot massage through clinical practice and by getting rid of the stale and taking in the fresh.

The authors, Beijing

CHAPTER 1   ANCIENT MASSAGE

I. Development of Traditional Hand and Foot Massage

Traditional hand and foot massage originated from diagnostics using the hand and foot in traditional Chinese medicine. In the early developmental stage of traditional Chinese medicine, it was already known that abnormal changes on the hand and foot might indicate pathological disturbance of the internal organs. As mentioned in *The Yellow Emperor's Canon of Medicine*, the earliest classical medical book, written by various authors between 475 BC to 221 BC: "A hot sensation in the palm indicates the presence of heat pathogens in the internal organs; A cold sensation in the palm indicates the presence of cold pathogens in the internal organs.... Patients with diseases of the small intestine due to attack of severe cold pathogens may have a hot sensation on the shoulder and between the little finger and index finger." So, as a part of traditional Chinese medicine, diagnosis using the hand and foot appeared as early as other components of ancient medicine.

After traditional Chinese medicine gradually developed into a complete medical system with its own theories, therapies, recipes and herbs, diagnosis by hand and foot was still very limited compared with the more advanced four diagnostic methods—observation, olfaction and auscultation, interrogation and palpation for general diagnosis. Because of neglect by classical medicine physicians with their traditional conservative attitude of superiority, diagnosis using the hand, foot and eye remained a minor branch of medicine and was not accepted and practiced by the majority of physicians and so failed to develop. According to fragmentary statements scattered in a few medical books, hand and foot diagnosis remained in its primitive stage until the Qing Dynasty.

Although diagnosis by hand and foot was overlooked in medicine, it found a place to be carried forward in traditional hand fortune-telling. As a matter of fact, the fortune-tellers made an important contribution to the development of diagnosis as well as hand and foot massage. In *Ma Yi Shen Xiang* (Linen Clothes Miraculous Fortune-telling), published in the period between AD 960 and AD 1127, the shape of the hand and foot, creases on the palmar and dorsal sides of the hand and their relationship to the maintenance of health by physical and breathing exercises were mentioned in detail, and the 72 types of palmar creases were summarized. This was the first book to accurately describe the shape and creases of the hand and foot in detail, although it also contained much superstitious material. However, its analysis of physical and mental health according to hand and foot variation is still informative and useful.

During the Song and Ming dynasties, the development of fortune-telling reached its zenith, and along with it diagnosis and treatment by hand and foot also matured. In ancient China it was believed that "fortune-tellers may be good physicians" because they had wide social contact and rich life experiences for studying the psychology of common people, and the chance to obtain knowledge of common diseases. Through their close contact with people, and analysis and explaination of their health and diseases, they earned the confidence of their clients. Their diagnostic techniques and hand and foot treatment increasingly improved and gained acceptance by their patients. This is how this methods were applied and spread among common people through the centuries.

In the Ming and Qing dynasties, traditional Chinese massage further developed and combined with the theory of meridians and acupoints. By application of traditional massage maneuvers, the five Shu (well, spring, stream, river and sea) acupoints on the hand, and on the foot below the elbow and knee joints, were frequently selected for massage in the treatment of diseases. After absorbing the experience of folk hand and foot massage, an independent medical branch—regular hand and foot massage—was established.

However, as with traditional massage itself, hand and foot massage was not widely accepted as an independent branch of medicine equal in importance to other branches. Only a few fragmentary statements in few books on pediatric Tuina (traditional massage) mentioned it. It was only applied and adopted by common people, instead of qualified physicians.

In the 1980s, following the renewed popularity of Qigong and the *Yi Jing* (*Book of Changes*), traditional hand and foot massage was also back in vogue. Superstitious activities such as hand fortune-telling and the diagnosis of disease by palmar creases, and predicting the future by palmar creases also became more fashionable for a time.

Since the introduction of reflective sole therapy from Hong Kong and Taiwan into the mainland of China, traditional hand and foot massage has become more and more attractive for clinical application.

The investigation of unconventional therapies has become a trend in the development of contemporary medicine. Hand and foot massage is simple and easy to learn and practise, and effective in obtaining good therapeutic result. Therefore, as a treasure of traditional Chinese medicine, it will surely attract more attention around the world and again bring its benefits to mankind.

II. Concepts and Characteristics of Hand and Foot Massage

Hand and foot massage applies various kinds of stimulation

to acupoints or reflecting areas on the hand and foot specifically related to the internal organs and tissues. It is applied by physicians or the patients themselves to affect and adjust the functions of the corresponding organs and tissues. This therapy is based on the wholistic approach of traditional Chinese medicine and combines with the clinical experience of modern medicine. It produces stimulation transmitted from a superficial part to a deep part of the human body, and from a nearby part to a remote part. As a component of traditional Chinese medicine, this technique followed the development of general regular massage, was improved, developed, and gradually became established as an independent branch of medicine with unique and superior qualities.

The characteristics of hand and foot massage can be summarized as follows:

1. As an independent medical branch, hand and foot massage is easy to learn and practise, safe, comfortable, and produces good therapeutic results without harmful side effects. It can be used to treat and prevent diseases and maintain good health.

2. The local application of stimulation can adjust the functions of the entire body, reinforce the body's resistence, cure diseases, and prolong life. For prevention of diseases and maintenance of health, the manipulation must be gentle and applied regularly; and for the treatment of diseases, the manipulation should be heavier and even, and applied at the correct acupoints

and reflecting areas. The results obtained by local massage may be even better than those of the general massage.

3. This massage can be used along with other therapies to treat many diseases with good therapeutic results because it produces a generalized effect throughout the entire body. Together with medicinal treatment, patients can apply hand and foot massage themselves for the relief of many chronic illnesses.

4. Hand and foot massage should usually be applied symmetrically at acupoints on both sides of the body, so patients can easily remember the sequence for self-application. Self-massage may be applied at specific acupoints for different diseases according to the individual, the time, and the place. Several unsymmetrical acupoints can also be easily remembered and used in clinical application.

5. After the nature and function of the different acupoints and reflecting areas are learned and retained by the practitioner, he will be able to reasonably select and combine them for clinical use. Diagnosis using the hand and foot is also useful for preventing disease.

6. Herbal bath, herbal moxibustion, and the external application of herbal preparations also can be used in combination before, during, or after hand and foot massage to improve its therapeutic effect.

III. Indications for Hand and Foot Massage

Hand and foot massage can cure diseases and maintain

health through keeping the potency of the meridians, adjusting Ying qi (nutrients) and Wei qi (defensive energy), promoting the circulation of qi and blood, and balancing Yin and Yang; and it can also enhance body resistance, expel pathogens, control inflammation and pain, relieve stagnation, and promote the repair and regeneration of tissue. Therefore, this massage can be used to treat many medical, traumatological, orthopedic, gynecological, pediatric, dermatological and ENT diseases; and it can also be used for cosmetic purposes. This is a therapy easy to learn and practise for people of any age or occupation; and it can be applied at any time or place, especially useful where medical facilities are poor.

Of course, hand and foot massage is not a miraculous remedy capable of curing all diseases, although it can be used to treat many diseases without toxic side effects. However, it cannot produce apparent effects in the treatment of many acute progressive diseases, severe pain, or hemorrhage. Other contraindications will be mentioned in the following chapters.

CHAPTER 2 ANATOMY AND LOCATION OF ACUPOINTS AND REFLECTING AREAS ON HAND AND FOOT

I. Anatomy, Acupoints and Reflecting Areas of Hand

1. Anatomy of the hand:

The fantastic structure and nature of the hand is not well known to most people or even most scientists, although it is the part of the body most frequently used.

The human hand is a tool that has evolved along with the brain and is closely correlated with it. The dexterous structure of the human hand is the most advanced among all creatures.

People should become familiar with their hands. In normal humans the hand is composed of 27 bones. There are 8 carpal bones including the scaphoid, lunate, triangular, pisiform, greater and lesser trapezium, capitate and hamate bones. They are connected together by ligaments to perform various delicate movements of the palm and fingers. The palm is composed of 5

metacarpal bones which are connected to the 5 fingers. The
thumb is composed of 2 phalangeal bones, and each of other 4
fingers is composed of 3 phalangeal bones, so there are 14 phalangeal bones in all. The phalangeal bones of a finger are numbered as first, second and third from the proximal to the distal
end of the finger. The first segment is also called the proximal
phalanx, and the third one is also called the distal phalanx. All
hand bones are connected by muscles, ligaments and fibrous
bundles to perform various delicate movements (Fig. 2-1).

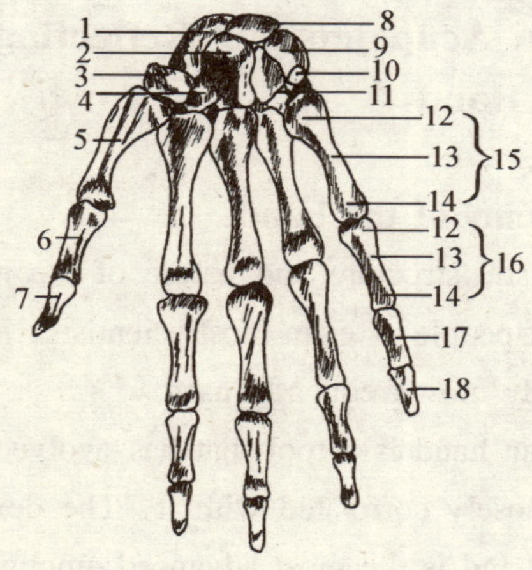

Fig. 2-1 Bones of the hand (palmar side)

1-scaphoid 2-cpitate 3-greater trapezium 4-lesser trapezium 5-first metacarpal 6-
proximal phalanx 7-distal phalanx 8-lunate 9-triangular 10-pisiform 11-hamate
12-base 13-body 14-caput 15-fifth metacarpal 16-first (proximal) phalax 17-sec-
ond (middle) phalanx 18-third (distal) phalax

The hand is innervated by the brain to carry out various

movements and is very sensitive to sensations constantly sending sensory nerve impulses to the brain. The hand can be divided into several layers including the skin, subcutaneous tissue, palmar aponeurosis, superficial palmar arch of blood vessels, nerves, tendons, deep palmar arch of blood vessels, metacarpal bones and interosseous muscles from superficial to the deepest layer. The palmar skin is covered with a thick layer of keratinized epithelium. The central part of the palmar skin is less movable because it is fixed by tense subcutaneous tissue and many fibrous septa, connected with the palmar aponeurosis. Thereby things can be held tightly in the hand. The palmar aponeurosis is a white, firm, triangular plate of dense connective tissue, tightly connected with the skin and subcutaneous tissue to assist wrist extension and finger flexibility. The hand is supplied with nuerous blood vessels and nerves. The superficial and deep palmar arches are mutually connected and send forth arterioles to supply nutrients to the parts of the hand. Although blood circulation through the superficial arch is blocked when something is held tightly in the hand, blood can still pass through the deep arch to the tips of the fingers without interfering with the blood supply to the rest of the hand. The nerves of the hand originate from the median, radial and ulnar nerves of the arm to innervate the hand muscles and skin. The numerous nerve endings gathered on the fingertips are very sensitive to pain and tactile sensations. There are many fibrous bundles in the subcutaneous tissue firmly connecting the skin of the distal phalanx with its periosteum. The central canaliculi of fibrous bundles are filled with fatty tissue and the arterioles passing through the fibrous bundles nourish the distal phalanx. The spaces in joints between the bones are filled with synovial fluid to facilitate nimble hand movement (Fig. 2-2).

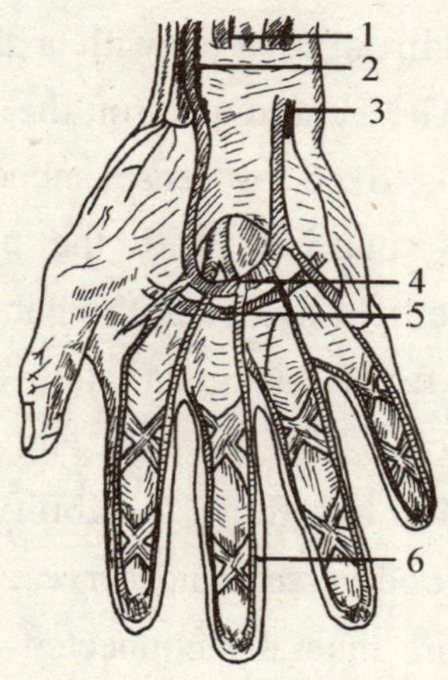

Fig. 2-2 Diagram of local anatomy of the palm
1-median nerve 2-radial artery, vein and nerve 3-ulnar artery, vein and nerve 4-superficial palmar arch 5-deep palmar arch 6-proper artery and nerve beside finger

The nails are a specific structure without sensory nerve endings (Fig. 2-3) and are attached to the distal phalanx with vital tissue at their base which shows the state of a person's health over a period of time. Therefore, it is useful indiagnostics since the color and shape of the nails can show sufficiency or deficiency of the nutrients being supplied to the limbs, as well as the condition of the entire body.

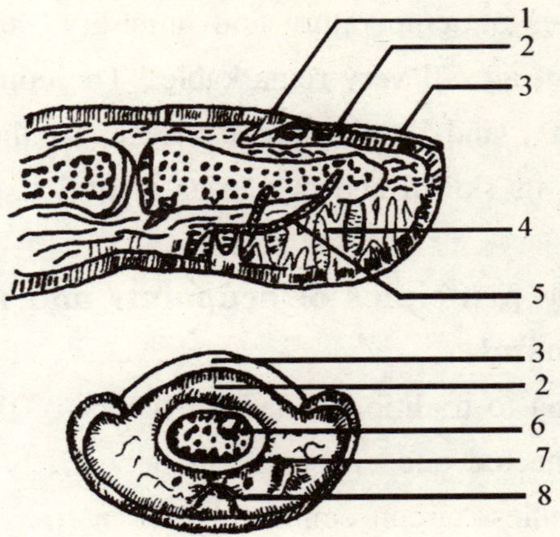

Fig. 2-3 Fingertips and nail structure

1-nail base 2-nail bed 3-nail 4-fibrous bundle 5-blood vessel of finger 6-phalangeal bone, 7-nerve 8-fibrous septum

The construction of the palm is compact, while the dorsal skin of the hand is thinner and its subcutaneous tissue is looser to allow flexible hand movement. The dorsum of the hand is arrayed with numerous veins and nerves to enable the hand to carry out its delicate functions.

With its complex structure the hand can performs various delicate and nimble movements under the control of the brain. According to experimental study, the hand shows a variation of cutaneous electrical activity similar to that of the brain. The mechanism of this similarity between the brain and hand is still unknown, but it demonstrates the specificity of the hand. The hand's tolerance for mechanical strain, its sensitivity to environmental changes of temperature and humidity, and its range of self-adjustment are all very remarkable. The complicated structure, functions, and physiological reflexes of the hand are the foundation of its skilful and dexterous activities.

2. Basic principles of acupoints and reflecting areas on the hand:

According to traditional medical theory of the meridian, a mutually connected and crisscrossing network is present in the body as an endless circuit connecting the internal organs and the external limbs. However, according to modern concepts this is a nervelike channel system, temporarily composed of cells, connecting the external and internal structures and adjusting the functions of the entire body. There are 12 regular meridians, and they originate from or stop at limb terminals. Six of these meridins are the hand meridians including the hand Taiyin lung, hand Yangming large intestine, hand Jueyin pericardium, hand Shaoyang triple energizer, hand Shaoyin heart, and hand Taiyang small intestine meridians. The acupoints and areas on the regular meridians are called regular acupoints, and there are 23 regular acupoints on the hand, 9 on the palm, and 14 on the dorsum of the hand.

With the development of medical practice, people discovered more and more acupoints and their specific therapeutic effects, although they are not located on the meridians. These are called extra acupoints, and there are 77 extra acupoints on the hand, increasing the available locations for the application of therapeutic stimulation.

In addition, another group of reflecting points and areas were proposed by some scholars and given the name holographic points and areas, derived from the idea of the biological holographic phenomenon. These scholars believed that there are local reflecting points on the body corresponding to each independent segment and part of the body. The first group of 12 holographic points was found beside the second metacarpal bone. At the same time, the holographic areas corresponding to different organs and tissues of the body were also found on the hand, and an apparent adjusting effect could be produced in the body by an application of massage to these areas. It seemed very interesting that they could independently produce effects similar to those produced by the regular and extra acupoints. And sometimes stimulation applied to these holographic areas could produce certain effects not reproducible by applying the same stimulation to acupoints located in the same areas. This indicated that the holographic area itself could independently produce different effects, although located in a same region as the acupoints. So we may propose the existence of a health record of the body, from certain developmental stages, retained in the living cells, and the existence of an adjusting mechanism capable of affecting the entire body by stimulating a very limited area.

The regular acupoints, extra acupoints, and holographic points and reflecting areas can be considered as independent "information-inducing units," and through them the adjusting impulse can be transmitted from the local point or area to the rest of the body. Scientific investigators may study the mechanism of this phenomenon if they are interested, but clinicians need only learn and master the acupoints and areas for clinical practice, without necessarily knowing the underlying reasons.

For the convenience of the reader, the proportional unit of the thumb width (Fig. 2-4) should be mentioned first.

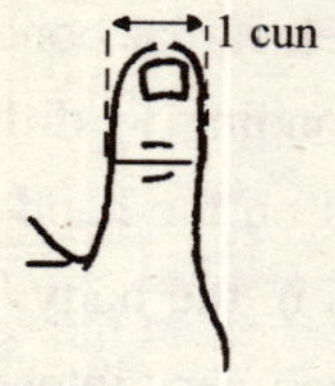

Fig. 2-4 The "Cun"

The unit of length used since ancient times for locating acupoints is called a "cun," which is equal to the width of the interphalangeal joint of the thumb. Therefore, the exact length of a cun varies from person to person. For convenience in clinical practice, the width of the physician's interphalangeal thumb joint may be used as a cun, if his physique is similar to that of his patient. One cun can be further divided into 10 fractions, and one-tenth of a cun is called one "fen."

3. Distribution of acupoints and areas on palmar side of the hand:

In this section, 9 regular and 34 extra acupoints, and 42 holographic areas are described as follows:

1) Regular acupoints:

（1）Taiyuan（LU 9）:

Location: At the radial end of palmar carpal crease and in a depression on the radial side of radial artery（Fig. 2-5）.

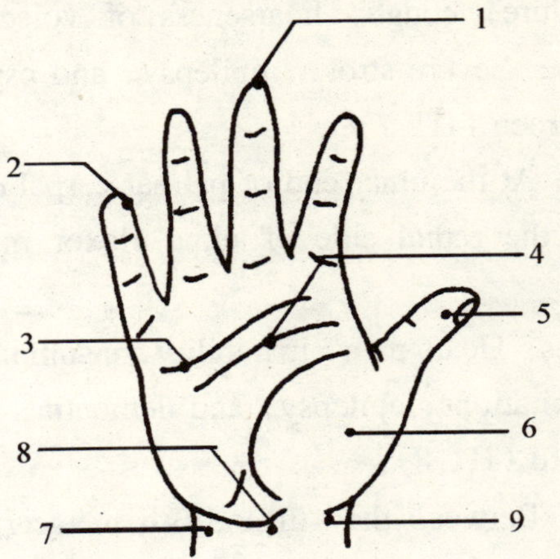

Fig. 2-5 Regular acupoints on palmar side of hand

1-Zhongchong（PC 9）2-Shaochong（HT 9）3-Shaofu（HT 8）4-Laogong（PC 8）5-Shaoshang（LU 11）6-Yuji（LU 10）7-Shenmen（HT 7）8-Daling（PC 7）9-Taiyuan（LU 9）

Indications: Cough, asthma, hemoptysis, chest pain, sore throat, wrist and arm pain, and pain and distension of breast.

（2）Yuji（LU 10）:

Location: Beside the midpoint of first metacarpal bone and on the dorso-palmar boundary of hand（Fig. 2-5）.

Indications: Cough, hemoptysis, sore throat, aphonia, fever, headache, chest pain, and pain in breast.

（3）Shaoshang（LU 11）:

Location: It is 0.1 cun beside the radial corner of thumb-nail (Fig. 2-5).

Indications: Sore throat, nasal bleeding, fever, coma, respiratory failure, cough, hoarseness of voice, swelling of cheek, syncope, severe stroke, epilepsy, and psychosis.

(4) Shenmen (HT 7):

Location: At the ulnar end of palmar carpal crease and in a depression on the radial side of ulnar flexor muscle of wrist (Fig. 2-5).

Indications: Heart pain, irritability, insomnia, poor memory, heart palpitations, epilepsy, and dementia.

(5) Shaofu (HT 8):

Location: Between the 4th and 5th metacarpal bones and on the crease passing through the center of palm; or at a spot between the 4th and 5th metacarpal bones where the tip of little finger just reaches when the hand is clenched in a fist (Fig. 2-5).

Indications: Heart palpitations, chest pain, spasm of little finger, vulvar itching, incontinence of urine, and difficult urination.

(6) Shangchong (HT 9):

Location: It is 0.1 cun beside the radial corner of nail of little finger (Fig. 2-5).

Indications: Heart palpitations, heart pain, febrile diseases, psychosis, coma, and pain and distension of chest and flanks.

(7) Daling (PC 7):

Location: At the midpoint of palmar carpal crease and between the tendons of long palmar muscle and radial flexor muscle of wrist (Fig. 2-5).

Indications: Hematemesis, restlessness, psychosis, heart pain, heart pacpitations, pain of wrist, unconsciousness, stomachache, vomiting, and pain of chest and flanks.

(8) Laogong (PC 8):

Location: At the midpoint of a palmar crease passing through the center of palm; or at a spot between 2nd and 3rd metacharpal bones where the tip of middle finger just reaches when the hand is clenched in a fist (Fig. 2-5).

Indications: Epilepsy, psychosis, hysteria, vomiting, foul odor in mouth, aphtha of mouth, hiccups, and hotness in palm.

(9) Zhongchong (PC 9):

Location: At the tip of middle finger (Fig. 2-5).

Indications: Coma, convulsions, night crying in babies, stiff tongue, heart pain, febrile diseases, and prodromal symptoms of stroke.

2) Extra acupoints:

(1) Shixuan acupoint (EX-PH 1):

Location: At all 10 fingertips and 0.1 cun from the edge of nail border (Fig. 2-6).

Indications: Coma, epilepsy, hysteria, high fever, con-

sions in children, and tonsillitis.

(2) Sifeng acupoint (EX-PH 2):

Locations: At the midpoint of palmar crease of proximal interphalangeal joint of index, middle, ring, and little fingers of both hands (Fig. 2-6).

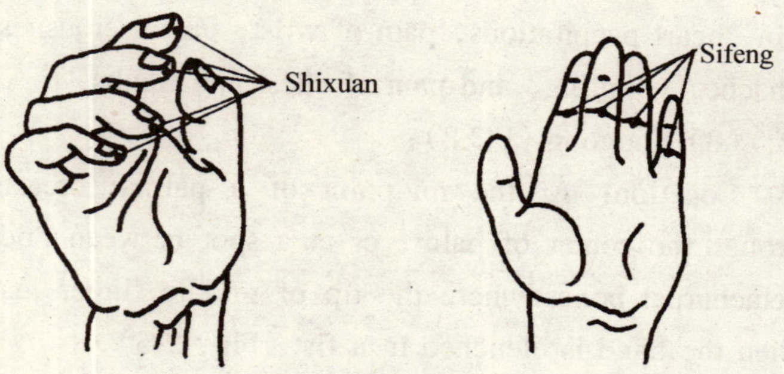

Fig. 2-6 Shixuan and Sifeng acupoints

Indications: Indigestive malnutrition and whooping cough.

(3) Endocrine acupoint (EX-PH 3):

Location: At the top of thenar prominence (Fig. 2-7).

Indications: It can be used to treat endocrinal diseases and adjust function of adrenal gland, thymus, and thyroid gland.

(4) Chest pain acupoint (EX-PH 4):

Location: At the radial border of interphalangeal joint of thumb and on the dorso-palmar boundary of hand (Fig. 2-7).

Indications: Contusion of chest, intercostal neuralgia, herpes zoster with chest pain, vomiting, diarrhea, and epilepsy.

(5) Uterus acupoint (EX-PH 5):

Location: At the midpoint between the junction of little fingers and the first distal palmar crease (Fig. 2-7).

Indications: Diseases of reproductive system including diseases of ovary, testis, and menstruation.

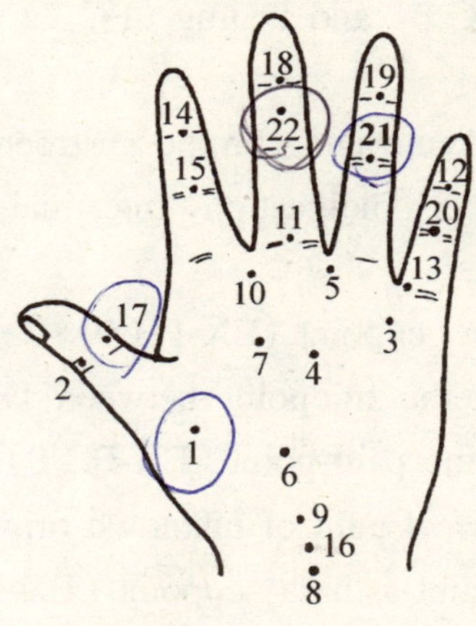

Fig. 2-7 Extra acupoints on palmar side of hand

1-endocrine 2-chest pain 3-uterus 4-hyperhidrosis 5-toothache 6-stomach and intestine pain 7-Laogong (PC 8) 8-Daling (PC 7) 9-heel pain 10-cough and asthma 11-oral aphtha 12-bed-wetting 13-heart palpitations 14-colon 15-urethra 16-anti-convulsion 17-spleen 18-heart 19-lung 20-Mingmen 21-liver 22-pelvic cavity

(6) Hyperhidrosis acupoint (EX-PH 6):

Location: At the center of palm (Fig. 2-7).

Indications: Hyperhidrosis and mental anxiety.

(7) Toothache acupoint (EX-PH 7):

Location: It is 1 cun proximal to the junction of middle

and ring fingers (Fig. 2-7).

Indications: Dull and continuous toothache.

(8) Stomach and intestine pain acupoint (EX-PH 8):

Location: Also called Xiaotianxin, it is at the midpoint between Laogong (PC 8) and Daling (PC 7) acupoints (Fig. 2-7).

Indications: Acute and chronic gastroenteritis, gastric and duodenal peptic ulcer, indigestion, intestinal ascaris, coma with fever, and rhinitis.

(9) Heel pain acupoint (EX-PH 9):

Location: At the midpoint between Daling (PC 7) and stomach and intestine pain point (EX-PH 8) (Fig. 2-7).

Indications: Heel pain of unknown origin.

(10) Cough and asthma acupoint (EX-PH 10):

Location: At the ulnar border of metacarpal joint of index finger (Fig. 7).

Indications: Acute and chronic bronchitis, bronchial asthma, and neurotic headache.

(11) Oral aphtha acupoint (EX-PH 11):

Location: At the midpoint of palmar crease of carpometacarpal joint of middle finger (Fig. 2-7).

Indications: Oral aphtha and oral ulcers.

(12) Bed-wetting acupoint (EX-PH 12):

Location: At the midpoint of palmar crease of distal interphalangeal joint of little finger (Fig. 2-7).

Indications: Not awakened by bed-wetting at night and frequent ruination.

(13) Heart palpitation acupoint (EX-PH 13):

Location: At the radial border of carpometacarpal joint of little finger (Fig. 2-7).

Indications: Heart palpitations, profuse menstrual discharge, and dysmenorrhea.

(14) Colon acupoint (EX-PH 14):

Location: At the midpoint of palmar crease of distal interphalangeal joint of index finger (Fig. 2-7).

Indications: Diseases of colon and rectum, such as colitis and hemorrhoids.

(15) Urethra acupoint (EX-PH 15):

Location: At the midpoint of palmar crease of proximal interphalangeal joint of index finger (Fig. 2-7).

Indications: Diseases of urethra, small intestine, and lower abdomen.

(16) Anti-convulsion acupoint (EX-PH 16):

Location: At the midpoint between thenar and hypothenar prominence (Fig. 2-7).

Indications: Convulsions due to high fever.

(17) Spleen acupoint (EX-PH 17):

Location: At the midpoint of palmar crease of interphalangeal joint of thumb (Fig. 2-7).

Indications: Diseases of spleen and stomach, edema due to accumulation of water, and spleen dysfunction.

(18) Heart acupoint (EX-PH 18):

...lar crease of distal inter-... dle finger (Fig. 2-7).

... diovascular system, such as ... of blood pressure, and bradycar-

... (EX-PH 19):

... e midpoint of palmar crease of distal inter-phal... ring finger (Fig. 2-7).

Indications: Diseases of respiratory system, such as upper respiratory infection, infection of lungs, and profuse sputum.

(20) Mingmen acupoint (EX-PH 20):

Location: At the midpoint of palmar crease of proximal interphalangeal joint of little finger (Fig. 2-7).

Indications: Diseases of reproductive system, such as oligomenorrhea, inactive sperm, and urinary tract infection.

(21) Liver acupoint (EX-PH 21):

Location: At the midpoint of palmar crease of proximal interphalangeal joint of ring finger (Fig. 2-7).

Indications: Diseases of liver and gallbladder, reduced bile excretion, and discomfort over liver region.

(22) Pelvic cavity acupoint (EX-PH 22):

Location: Also called Renzhongxin, it is at the midpoint between two interphalangeal creases of middle finger (Fig. 2-7).

Indications: Diseases of abdominal and pelvic cavity, such as discomfort, distension, pain and straining sensation in abdomen, adnexitis, and influenza.

(23) Hypothenar prominence acupoint (EX-PH 23):

Location: On the palmar side of hand on the radial border of 5th metacarpal bone and at the junction of its middle one-third and lower one-third, and at the midpoint of abductor muscle of little finger (Fig. 2-8).

Indications: Depressive and paranoic psychosis.

(24) Finger and palm acupoint (EX-PH 24):

Location: On the palmar side of hand, at the junction of middle and ring fingers, and nearer to the former (Fig. 2-8).

Indications: Insomnia, poor memory, epilepsy, and schizophrenia.

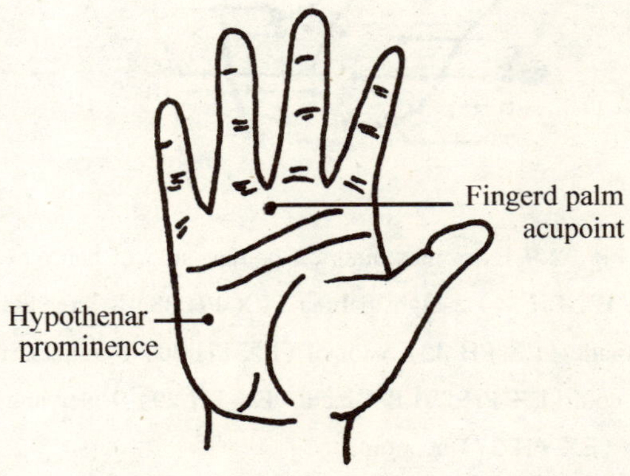

Fig. 2-8 Hypothenar prominence acupoint and finger and palm acupoint

(25) Common cold acupoint (EX-PH 25):

Location: Near the radial border of palm and 1 cun proximal to the base of first phalanx (Fig. 2-9).

Indications: Common cold, tosillitis, and toothache.

(26) Anti-tussive acupoint (EX-PH 26):

Location: On the radial border of palm and 5 fen proximal to the depression behind the base of first metacarpal bone (Fig. 2-9).

Indications: Cough, shortness of breath, and rheumatic heart disease.

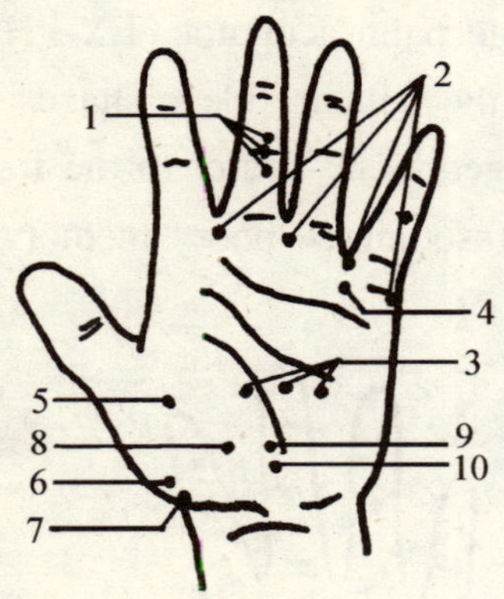

Fig. 2-9 Extra acupoints on palmar side of hand

1-Neizhongkui (EX-PH 34) 2-eight palmar (EX-PH 33) 3-three Jianli (EX-PH 31) 4-anti-asthmatic (EX-PH 32) 5-tonsil (EX-PH 30) 6-anti-tussive (EX-PH 26) 7-common cold (EX-PH 25) 8-Yinchi (EX-PH 29) 9-Neiyangchi (EX-PH 28) 10-Banmen (EX-PH 27) acupoint

(27) Banmen acupoint (EX-PH 27):

Location: It is 5 fen distal to the midpoint of wrist palmar crease (Fig. 2-9).

Indications: Diseases of small intestine, triple energizer,

and lungs.

(28) Neiyangchi acupoint (EX-PH 28):

Location: It is 1 cun distal to the midpoint of wrist palmar crease (Fig. 2-9).

Indications: Stomatitis and tinea unguium.

(29) Yinchi acupoint (EX-PH 29):

Location: On the radial side of Neiyangchi acupoint (EX-PH 28) and 1 cun from it (Fig. 2-9).

Indications: Hemoptysis and laryngitis.

(30) Tonsil acupoint (EX-PH 30):

Location: On the thenar prominence on the ulnar border of first metacarpal bone and at the midpoint of this bone (Fig. 2-9).

Indications: Tonsillitis and laryngitis.

(31) Three Jianli acupoints (EX-PH 31):

Location: They are in the central area of palm; one acupoint is 1 cun proximal to the midpoint of the interosseous space between 3rd and 4th metacarpal bones, and the other two acupoints are 5 fen on either side of the first acupoint (Fig. 2-9).

Indications: Diseases of liver and spleen, headache, eye diseases, bronchitis, bronchial asthma, heart palpitations, heart failure, and nephritis.

(32) Anti-asthmatic acupoint (EX-PH 32):

Location: Between the capitula of 4th and 5th metacarpal bones (Fig. 2-9).

Indications: Chronic senile bronchitis and asthma.

(33) Eight palmar acupoints (EX-PH 33):

Location: On each hand there are 3 acupoints 2 fen proximal to the midpoint of the web border between index and middle fingers, middle and ring fingers, and ring and little fingers respectively, and one other acupoint is 2 fen proximal to the ulnar end of palmar crease of 5th carpometacarpal joint (Fig. 2-9).

Indications: Redness and swelling of palm, paralysis of fingers, distension and pain of eyeball, and bed-wetting.

(34) Neizhongkui acupoints (EX-PH 34):

Location: One of the 3 acupoints is at the midpoint of the palmar proximal interphalangeal crease of middle finger, and the other 2 acupoints are 1 fen, distal and proximal respectively, to the first acupoint (Fig. 2-9).

Indication: Psoriasis.

3) Holographic points and reflecting areas:

(1) Holographic points:

According to the biological holographic theory, a group of holographic points correspondent to the human body is present in each independent part of the body. For example, a group of biological holographic points is present in each phalanx and metacarpal bone of the hand. Each group of holographic points is divided by Professor Zhang Yingqing into 12 points correspendent to the head, neck, arm, lung and heart, liver, stomach, duodenum, kidney, waist, and leg and foot, arranged from distal end to proximal end (Fig. 2-10). The distal end in a body part is the head point, and the proximal end is the foot

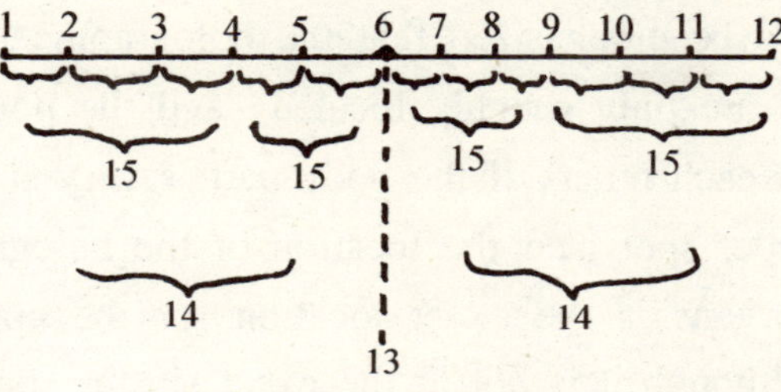

Fig. 2-10 Arrangement of biological holographic points
1-head 2-neck 3-arm 4-lung and heart 5-liver 6-stomach 7-duodenum 8-kidney
9-waist 10-lower abdomen 11-leg 12-foot 13-midpoint 14-two divisions 15-three
divisions

point; the midpoint between them is the stomach point; the midpoint between the head point and the stomach point is the point lung and heart point; the distance between the head point and the lung and heart point is divided into three equal portions. The distal dividing point is for the neck, and the proximal dividing point is for the arm point; the midpoint between the lung and heart point and stomach point is the liver point; the midpoint between the stomach point and the foot point is the waist point; the distance between the stomach point and the waist point is divided into three equal portions. The distal dividing point is for the duodenum and the proximal dividing point is for the kidney. And the distance between the waist point and the foot point is also divided into three equal portions; the distal dividing point is for the lower abdomen and the proximal dividing point is for the leg.

It should be emphasized that the holographic points mentioned above are only roughly located, and the points may be very close to each other, if the body part is very short. Therefore, the tender spot near the location of the holographic point for certain organs is the exact location for the application of treatment, although it is not at the exact site as shown in Fig. 2-10. A miniature of the whole body is set into a part with the head at the distal end and the foot at the proximal end. The important structures of the body may be arranged in sequence in the miniature.

(2) Holographic reflecting areas:

The holographic reflecting areas correspondent to the related organs arrayed over the palm are discovered through continuous clinical practice and the accumulation of clinical experience. Stimulation at those reflecting areas can adjust the function of their related organs to maintain health and treat diseases. The reflecting areas are named after their related organs, or by the specific diseases curable by stimulating them. The common holographic reflecting areas are shown in Fig. 2-11.

As with the application of holographic points, the location of holographic reflecting areas can be remembered by following the principle of their arrangement, and the reflecting areas should be flexibly selected for use. Regular and even stimulation applied at the more sensitive spots will produce the best therapeutic results.

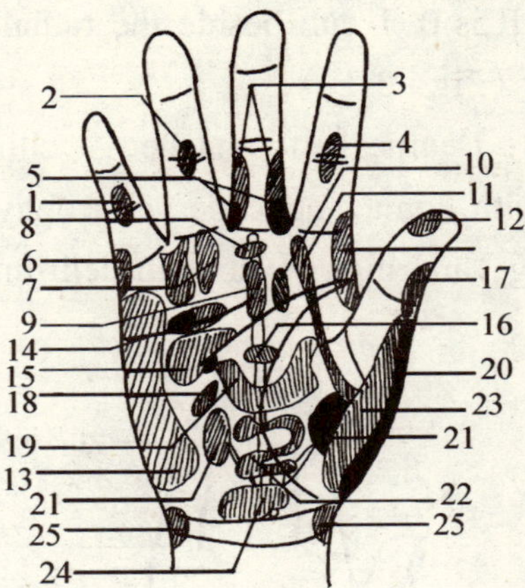

Fig. 2-11 Holographic reflecting areas on palmar side of hand

1-urogenital organs 2-adjustment of liver and gallbladder 3-ear 4-adjustment of lower abdomen 5-eye 6-shoulder 7-lung 8-mouth 9-esophagus 10-diabetes mellitus zone 11-cancer zone 12-brain 13-lymphatic immunity zone (lower body to upper body) 14-breast 15-liver and gallbladder 16-pancreas 17-head and neck 18-spleen 19-stomach 20-spinal column (neck to sacrum) 21-waist and kidney 22-intestine 23-heart and chest 24-reproduction 25-reproductive gland

4. Distribution of acupoints and reflecting areas on dorsal side of the hand

There are 14 regular acupoints, 43 extra acupoints, and 24 holographic points and reflecting areas on the dorsal side of the hand as follows:

1) Regular acupoints:

(1) Shangyang (LI 1):

Location: It is 0.1 cun beside the radial corner of nail of the index finger (Fig. 2-12).

Indications: Deafness, toothache, swelling of cheek, sore throat, stroke with coma, optic nerve atrophy, febrile diseases without sweating, and high fever with delirium.

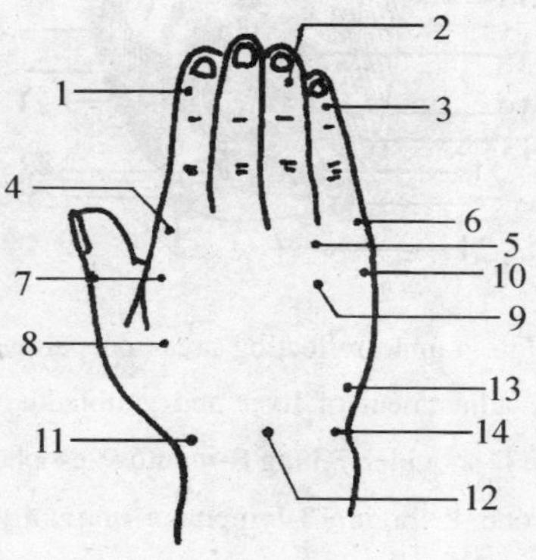

Fig. 2-12 Regular acupoints on dorsal side of hand

1-Shangyang (LI 1) 2-Guanchong (TE 1) 3-Shaoze (SI 1) 4-Erjian (LI 2) 5-Yemen (TE 2) 6-Qian'gu (SI 2) 7-Sanjian (LI 3) 8-Hegu (LI 4) 9-Zhongzhu (TE 3) 10-Houxi (SI 3) 11-Yangxi (LI 5) 12-Yangchi (TE 4) 13-Wan'gu (SI 4) 14-Yanggu (SI 5)

(2) Sanjian (LI 3):

Location: In a depression proximal to the capitulum of 2nd metacarpal bone and on its radial side when the hand is clenched in a fist (Fig. 2-12).

Indications: Toothache on lower jaw, sore throat, redness and swelling of dorsum of hand, gum swelling and pain, eye pain, nasal bleeding, fever, fullness in chest, increase of intestinal gurgling, constipation or diarrhea.

(3) Erjian (LI 2):

Location: In a depression distal to the capitulum of metacarpal bone of index finger and on its radial side when the hand is clenched in a fist (Fig. 2-12).

Indications: Blurred vision, nasal bleeding, toothache, swelling of cheek, deviation of mouth and eye, sore throat, febrile diseases, food stagnation, and constipation.

(4) Hegu (LI 4):

Location: Between the 1st and 2nd metacarpal bones and beside the midpoint of radial border of the 2nd bone, or at the top of prominence of muscle lump between 1st and 2nd metacarpal bones. The palmar crease of the interphalangeal joint of the thumb of one hand is put on the web border between thumb and index finger of the other hand and the tip of the first thumb reaches this acupoint as the interphalangeal joint is flexed (Fig. 2-12).

Indications: Febrile diseases, headache, toothache, lockjaw, deviation of mouth, nasal bleeding, deafness, sore throat, amenorrhea, prolonged labor, abdominal pain, spasm, arm pain, convulsion in children, hypertension, paralysis of arm, Bi-syndrome, psychosis, and epilepsy.

(5) Yangxi (LI 5):

Location: On the radial end of dorsal crease of wrist and in a depression between short and long extensor muscles of thumb

(Fig. 2-12).

Indications: Headache, red eye, deafness, toothache, and pain and swelling of wrist joint.

(6) Shaoze (SI 1):

Location: It is 0.1 cun beside the ulnar corner of the nail of little finger (Fig. 2-12).

Indications: Milky eye, sore throat, stroke with coma, febrile diseases, oligogalactia after childbirth, red and swollen tongue, and headache.

(7) Qian'gu (SI 2):

Location: It is at the ulnar end of the crease of 5th metacarpophalangeal joint when the hand is clenched in a fist and on the dorsopalmar boundary (Fig. 2-12).

Indications: Febrile diseases, headache, eye pain, sore throat, numbness of fingers, deafness, red and swollen tongue, pain and swelling of cheek, chest distress, and failure to lactate after childbirth.

(8) Houxi (SI 3):

Location: In a depression proximal to the 5th metacarpophalangeal joint when the hand is clenched in a fist and on the dorsopalmar boundary (Fig. 2-12).

Indications: Headache, stiff neck, pain of back and waist, psychosis, malaria, deafness, milky eye, nasal bleeding, toothache on upper jaw, spasms and pain in elbow and arm, and spasms in fingers.

(9) Wan'gu (SI 4):

Location: On the dorsal side of hand and in a depression formed by base of 5th metacarpal, pisiform and hamate bones (Fig. 2-12).

Indications: Febrile diseases, jaundice, spasms in fingers, wrist pain, headache, tinnitus, and pain in shoulder, arm and nape.

(10) Yanggu (SI 5):

Location: On the ulnar side of wrist joint and in a depression distal to the capitulum of ulna bone (Fig. 2-12).

Indications: Swelling of neck and chin, tinnitus, deafness, psychosis, convulsions, febrile diseases, pain of lateral side of arm, stiff tongue, lockjaw, and eye pain.

(11) Guanchong (TE 1):

Location: It is 0.1 cun beside the ulnar corner of nail of ring finger (Fig. 2-12).

Indications: Headache, red eye, sore throat, febrile diseases, irritability, and stiffness and pain of tongue.

(12) Zhongzhu (TE 3):

Location: In a depression proximal to and between the capitula of 4th and 5th metacarpal bones when the hand is clenched in a fist (Fig. 2-12).

Indications: Tinnitus, deafness, migraine, stiff neck, red eye, sore throat, febrile diseases, pain in fingers with difficult extension, malaria, and redness, swelling and pain in hand and arm.

(13) Yemen (TE 2):

Location: In a depression distal to and between the carpophalangeal joints of ring and little fingers when the hand is clenched in a fist (Fig. 2-12).

Indications: Migraine, red eye, deafness, sore throat, malaria, and pain in hand and arm.

(14) Yangchi (TE 4):

Location: On the dorsal crease of wrist and in a depression on the ulnar border of common extensor muscle of fingers (Fig. 2-12).

Indications: Wrist, shoulder, and back pain, malaria, lumbago, diabetes mellitus, redness and swelling of ear auricle, deafness, and tinnitus.

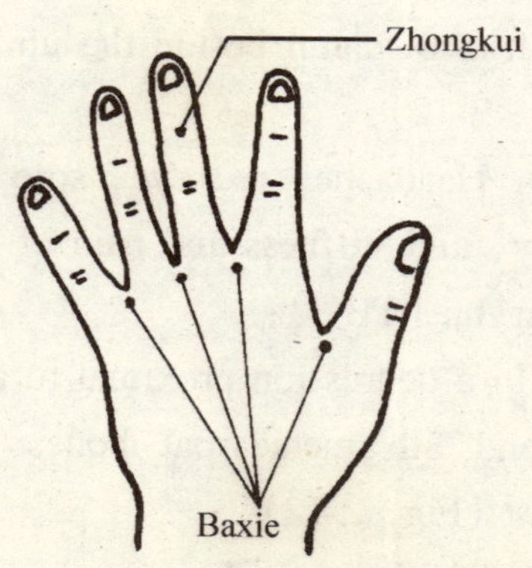

Fig. 2-13 Zhongkui and Baxie acupoints

2) Extra acupoints:

(1) Zhongkui acupoint (EX-DH 1):

Location: At the midpoint of dorsal crease of proximal interphalangeal joint of middle finger (Fig. 2-13).

Indications: Dysphagia and vomiting (moxibustion allowed).

(2) Baxie acupoints (EX-DH 2):

Location: They are on the dorsopalmar boundary of hand between each pair of neighboring fingers, on both hands, 8 in all (Fig. 2-13).

Indications: Fever with irritability, eye pain, swelling and pain in dorsum of hand, and poisonous snake bite.

(3) Waist and leg pain acupoints (EX-DH 3):

Location: They are 1.5 cun distal to the dorsal crease of wrist, one on the radial side of tendon of extensor muscle of index finger and another one on the ulnar side of tendon of extensor muscle of ring finger, 2 points on each hand; the first is called Weiling, and the second is called Jingling in Tuina (traditional massage) for children (Fig. 2-14a).

Indications: Sprain, rheumatism and strain with acute or chronic pain in waist and leg (better for acute attack in waist), sudden death of children due to convulsions, coma, asthma with phlegm and whistling, vomiting without vomitus, indigestive malnutrition, and pterygium.

(4) Arthralgia acupoint (EX-DH 4a, 4b, 4c and 4d):

Location: This is a group of acupoints arrayed near the dorsopalmar boundary of the hand. The elbow pain acupoint is at the midpoint of palmar crease of metacarpophalangeal joint of thumb（EX-DH 4d, Fig. 2-14b）; the knee pain acupoint（EX-DH 4a）is at the midpoint of dorsal crease of metacarpophalangeal joint of thumb; the ankle pain acupoint（EX-DH 4b）is on the radial side of metacarpophalangeal joint of thumb and on the dorsopalmar boundary of the hand; and the shoulder pain acupoint（EX-DH 4c）is on the radial side of metacarpophalangeal joint of index finger and on the dorsopalmar boundary of the hand（Fig. 2-14a）.

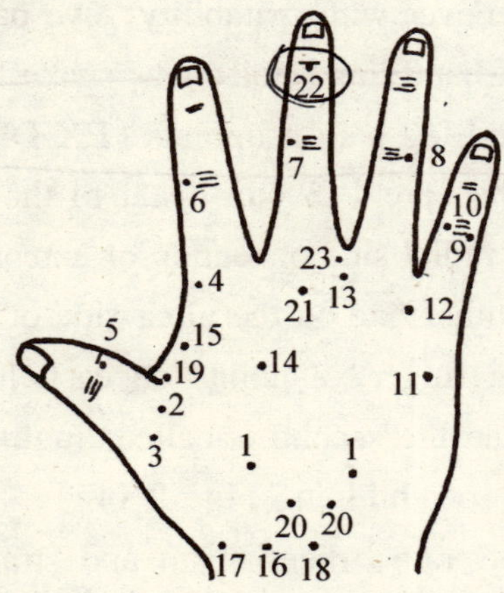

Fig. 2-14a Extra acupoints on dorsal side of hand

1-waist and leg pain 2-knee pain 3-ankle pain 4-shoulder pain 5-eye pain 6-frontal headache 7-parietal headache 8-temporal headache 9-occipital headache 10-perineal pain 11-spine pain 12-sciatic neuralgia 13-sore throat 14-stiff neck 15-nasal bleeding 16-hypertensing 17-Yangxi（LI 5）18-Yangchi（TE 4）19-brain 20-throracic spine pain 21-hypotensing 22-diaphragm 23-diarrhea

Indications: Pain of various joints due to rheumatism or

sprain.

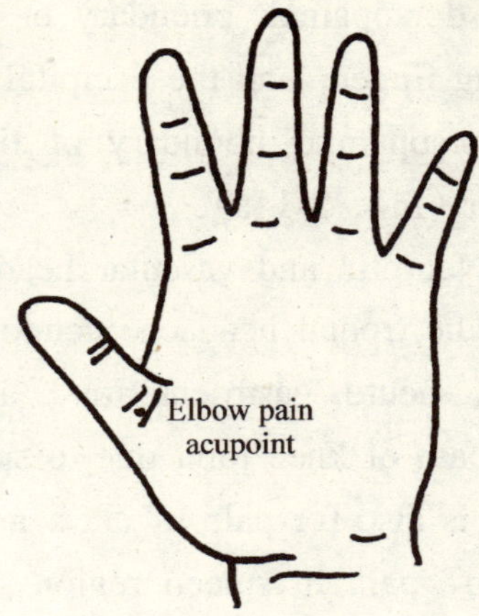

Fig. 2-14b Elbow pain acupoint

(5) Eye pain acupoint (EX-DH 5):

Location: On the ulnar side of interphalangeal joint of thumb and on the dorsopalmar boundary of the hand (Fig. 2-14a).

Indications: Acute conjunctivitis, kerotitis, sty, and glaucoma with eye pain.

(6) Headache acupoints (EX-DH 6a, 6b, 6c and 6d):

Location: This is a group of acupoints arrayed on the dorsopalmar boundary. The frontal headache acupoint is on the radial dorsopalmar boundary of proximal interphalangeal joint of index finger; the parietal headache acupoint is on the radial dorsopalmar boundary of proximal interphalangeal joint of middle finger; the temporal headache acupoint is on the dorsopalmar boundary of ulnar dorsopalmar boundary of proximal interphalangeal joint of ring finger; and the occipital headache acupoint is on the ulnar dorsopalmar boundary of first interphalangeal joint of little finger (Fig. 2-14a).

Indications: Neurotic and vascular headache at the correspondent region. The frontal headache acupoint is also for gastrointestinal colic, acute gastroenteritis, acute appendicitis, rheumatism, and pain of knee joint due to sprain; the temporal headache acupoint is also for pain of chest and flanks, discomfort of liver region, pain in spleen region, biliary colic, and costal neuralgia; and the occipital headache acupoint is also for acute tonsillitis, arm pain, redness and swelling of cheek, and hiccups.

(7) Perineal pain acupoint (EX-DH 7):

Location: On the radial dorsopalmar boundary of proximal interphalangeal joint of little finger (Fig. 2-14a).

Indications: Perineal pain and pain of external genital organs due to infection.

(8) Spine pain acupoint (EX-DH 8):

Location: On the ulnar dorsopalmar boundary of carpometacarpal joint of little finger (Fig. 2-14a).

Indications: Acute sprain of interspinous ligament, pain of coccyx, nasal obstruction, tinnitus, and lumbago due to herniation of intervertebral disc. It is chiefly used for pain of lumbar and sacral regions.

(9) Sciatic Neuralgia acupoint (EX-DH 9):

Location: On the dorsal side of hand and between the 4th and 5th carpometacarpal joints, but closer to the former (Fig. 2-14a).

Indications: Sciatic Neuralgia and pain in hip region.

(10) Sore throat acupoint (EX-DH 10):

Location: On the dorsal side of hand and between the 3rd and 4th carpometacarpal joints, but closer to the former (Fig. 2-14a).

Indications: Acute tonsillitis, acute pharyngitis, and trigeminal neuralgia.

(11) Stiff neck acupoint (EX-DH 11):

Location: On the dorsal side of hand and between the 2nd and 3rd carpometacarpal joints, 0.5 cun proximal to the former (Fig. 2-14a).

Indications: Stiff neck, sprain of neck and nape, and shoulder and arm pain.

(12) Nasal bleeding acupoint (EX-DH 12):

Location: At the midpoint of edge of web folding between thumb and index finger and on the dorsopalmar boundary (Fig. 2-14a).

Indication: Nasal bleeding.

(13) Hypertensing acupoint (EX-DH 13):

Location: On the dorsal crease of wrist and at the midpoint between Yangchi (TE 4) and Yangxi (LI 5) acupoints (Fig. 2-14a).

Indications: Hypotension due to various causes, rheumatism and sprain with swelling and pain of wrist joint, and numbness and spasms in forearm.

(14) Brain acupoint (EX-DH 14):

Location: On the ulnar side of metacarpophalangeal joint of thumb (Fig. 2-14a).

Indications: Headache, dizziness, and poor memory.

(15) Thoracic spine pain acupoints (EX-DH 15).

Location: These are two acupoints in a depression distal to the crease of wrist and beside the tendon of extensor muscle of middle finger (Fig. 2-14a).

Indications: Pain over the thoracic spine, shoulder, and back.

(16) Hypotensing acupoint (EX-DH 16):

Location: On the dorsal side of hand and in the center of a depression over the metacarpophalangeal joint of middle finger when it is extended (Fig. 2-14a).

Indication: Hypertension.

(17) Diaphragm acupoint (EX-DH 17):

Location: At the midpoint of dorsal crease of distal interphalangeal joint of middle finger (Fig. 2-14a).

Indication: Hiccups due to spasms of diaphragm.

(18) Diarrhea acupoint (EX-DH 18):

Location: It is on the dersal side of hand, 1 cun distal to the junction of metacarpophalangeal joints of middle and ring fingers (Fig. 2-14a).

Indications: Diarrhea and tenesmus.

(19) Yiwofeng acupoint (EX-DH 19):

Location: On the dorsal crease of wrist and at the promixal end of 3rd metacarpal bone (Fig. 2-15).

Indications: Acute and chronic convulsions, diarrhea, and anal pain.

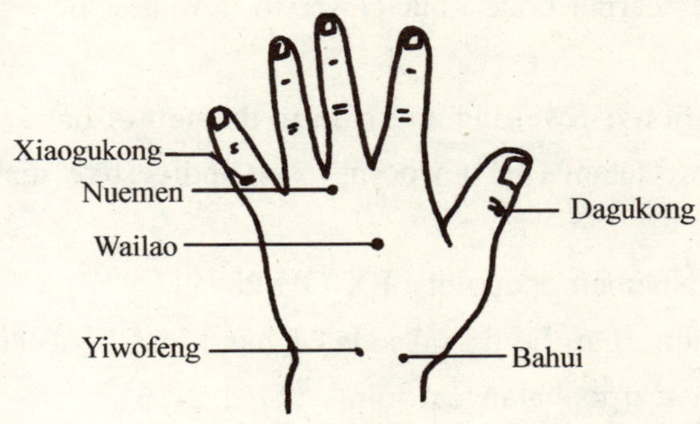

Fig. 2-15 Extra acupoints on dorsal side of hand

(20) Dagukong acupoint (EX-DH 20):

Location: On the dorsal side of thumb and at the center of its interphalangeal joint; and at the tip of this joint when the thumb is flexed (Fig. 2-15).

Indications: Eye diseases, vomiting, diarrhea, and nasal bleeding.

(21) Xiaogukong acupoint (EX-DH 21):

Location: On the dorsal side of little finger and at the tip of its proximal interphalangeal joint when the finger is flexed

(Fig. 2-15).

Indications: Various eye diseases, deafness, and pain in joints of little finger.

(22) Wailaogong (outer Laogong) acupoint (EX-DH 22):

Location: At the center of dorsum of hand between 2nd and 3rd metacarpal bone, but closer to the latter bone (Fig. 2-15).

Indications: Swelling and pain in dorsum of hand, paralysis of fingers, tetanus in newborns, and indigestive malnutrition in children.

(23) Nuemen acupoint (EX-DH 23):

Location: On the dorsal side of hand and between the 3rd and 4th metacarpophalangeal joints (Fig. 2-15).

Indication: Malaria.

(24) Bahui acupoint (EX-DH 24):

Location: It is on the dorsal side of hand, 5 fen distal to Yangxi (LI 5, Fig. 2-15).

Indications: Psychosis and epilepsy.

(25) Shanghegu (upper Hegu) acupoint (EX-DH 25):

Location: On the dorsal side of hand and in a depression distal to the bases of 1st and 2nd metacarpal bones (Fig. 2-16).

Indication: Toothache.

(26) Honggong acupoint (EX-DH 26):

Location: On the dorsal side of hand and in a depression distal to the bases of 2nd and 3rd metacarpal bones (Fig. 2-16).

Indications: External trauma of waist and limbs.

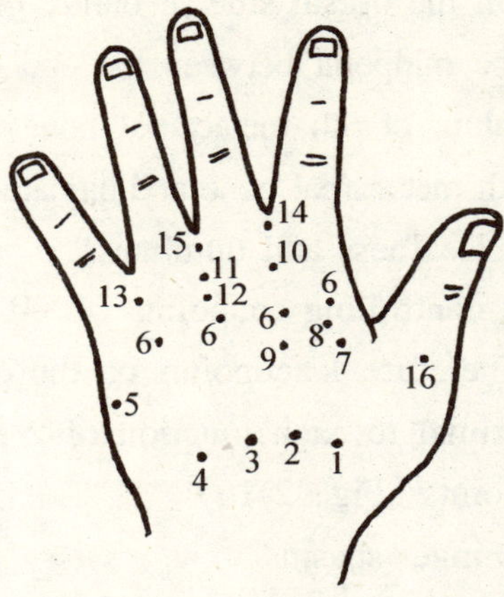

Fig. 2-16 Extra acupoints on dorsal side of hand

1-Shanghegu (EX-DH 25) 2-Honggong (EX-DH 26) 3-Hongyang (EX-DH 27) 4-Yonghong (EX-DH 28) 5-Shanghouxi (EX-DH 29) 6-spasm controlling 7-numbness 8-Hubian (EX-DH 32) 9-Yinmen (EX-DH 33) 10-Chaqi (EX-DH 34) 11-Kongji (EX-DH 35) 12-Tongling (EX-DH 36) 13-Chayi (EX-DH 37) 14-sprain 1 15-sprain 2 and 16-Hujincun (EX-DH 40) acupoints

(27) Hongyang acupoint (EX-DH 27):

Location: On the dorsal side of hand and in a depression distal to the bases of 3rd and 4th metacarpal bones (Fig. 2-16).

Indications: External trauma of chest and limbs.

(28) Yonghong acupoint (EX-DH 28):

Location: On the dorsal side of hand, in a depression distal to the bases of 4th and 5th metacarpal bones (Fig. 2-16).

Indications: External trauma and pain of waist and limbs.

(29) Shanghouxi (upper Houxi) acupoint (EX-DH 29):

Location: On the dorsal side of hand, on the ulnar border of hand and at the midpoint between the end of a palmar crease proximal to capitulum of 5th metacarpal bone and the depression between base of 5th metacarpal bone and hamate bone (Fig. 2-16).

Indications: Deafness and dumbness.

(30) Spasm-controlling acupoints (EX-DH 30):

Location: There are 4 acupoints on the dorsal side of each hand, 1 cun proximal to each junction of 2 neighboring metacarpophalangeal joints (Fig. 2-16).

Indication: Finger spasms.

(31) Numbness acupoint (EX-DH 31):

Location: On the dorsal side of hand, 0.15 cun beside the midpoint of radial border of 2nd metacarpal bone (Fig. 2-16).

Indications: Colic of stomach and numbness of index finger.

(32) Hubian acupoint (EX-DH 32):

Location: On the dorsal side of hand, slightly distal to the midpoint of radial border of 2nd metacarpal bone and 1.5 cun from the metacarpophalangeal joint (Fig. 2-16).

Indications: Schizophrenia, epilepsy, and hysteria.

(33) Yinmen acupoint (EX-DH 33):

Location: On the dorsal side of hand, at the center of the interosseous space between 2nd and 3rd metacarpal bones (Fig. 2-16).

Indications: Rheumatic arthritis of fingers and fingers sprain.

(34) Chaqi acupoint (EX-DH 34):

Location: On the dorsal side of hand, 5 fen proximal to a depression proximal to the capitula of 2nd and 3rd metacarpal bones (Fig. 2-16).

Indications: Stomach spasms and hypertension.

(35) Kongji acupoint (EX-DH 35):

Location: On the dorsal side of hand, 5 fen proximal to a depression proximal to the capitula of 3rd and 4th metacarpal bones (Fig. 2-16).

Indications: Intercostal neuralgia, stomachache, cholecystitis, ascaris in biliary tract, cholelithiasis, and pleuritis.

(36) Tongling acupoint (EX-DH 36):

Location: This is 5 fen distal to Kongji acupoint (EX-DH 35) (Fig. 2-16).

Indications: Toothache and chest pain.

(37) Chayi acupoint (EX-DH 37):

Location: Between the distal border of 4th and 5th metacarpophalangeal joints (Fig. 2-16).

Indications: Pleuritis and intercostal neuralgia.

(38) Sprain 1 acupoint (EX-DH 38):

Location: It is on the web border between index and middle fingers (Fig. 2-16).

Indication: Shoulder and upper limb sprain.

(39) Sprain 2 acupoint (EX-DH 39):

Location: On the web border between middle and ring fingers (Fig. 2-16).

Indications: Waist and lower limb sprain.

(40) Hujincun acupoint (EX-DH 40):

Location: On the dorsal side of thumb and at the center of its metacarpophalangeal joint (Fig. 2-16).

Indications: Sprain and rheumatic arthritis.

(41) Shousixue acupoints (EX-DH 41):

Location: These are 4 points, each is 1 fen beside the radial corner of free edge of nails of thumb and middle fingers on each hand (Fig. 2-17).

Indication: Food poisoning.

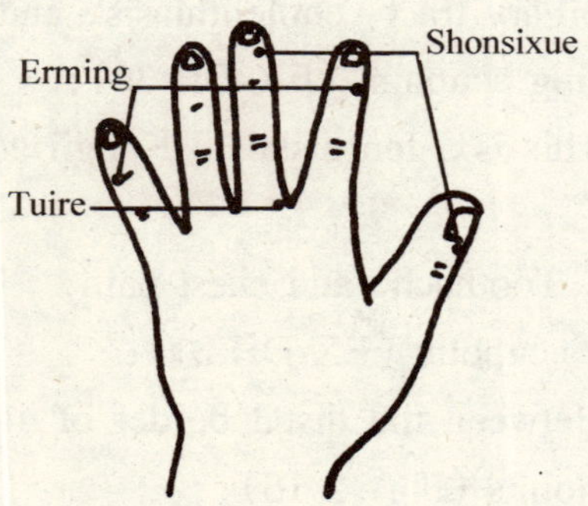

Fig. 2-17 Shousixue, Erming, and anti-febrile Tuire acupoints

(42) Erming acupoints (EX-DH 42):

Location: One of these 2 acupoints is on the ulnar end of dorsal crease of distal interphalangeal joint of little finger, the other is on the radial end of dorsal crease of distal interphalangeal joint of index finger (Fig. 2-17).

Indication: Eye diseases.

(43) Anti-febrile acupoint (EX-DH 43):

Location: On the dorsal side of hand, on the w
between index and middle fingers, and closer to the latter finger
(Fig. 2-17).

Indications: Fever and eye diseases.

3) Holographic points and reflecting areas:

(1) Biological holographic points:

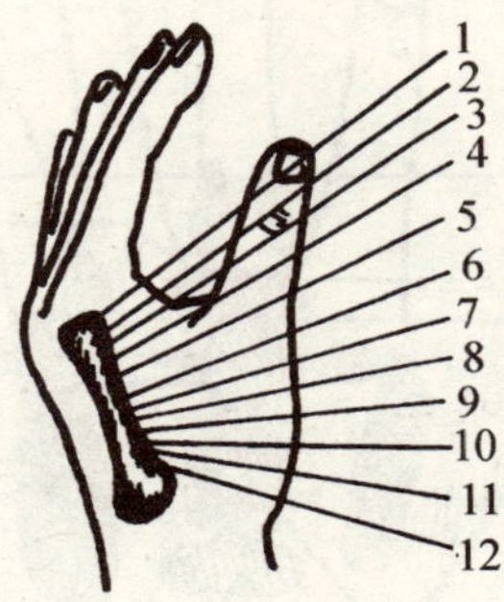

Fig. 2-18 Biological holographic points beside 2nd metacapal bone

1-head 2-neck 3-arm 4-lung and heart 5-liver 6-stomach 7-duodenum 8-kidney
9-waist 10-lower abdomen 11-leg 12-foot

The holographic points beside the 2nd metacarpal bone
(Fig. 2-18) are the most commonly used group of holographic
points, arranged in a sequence already mentioned in the holographic points on palmar side of hand. They can produce good
therapeutic results, in the treatment of their correspondent or-

gans or other structures on the same anatomical segment.

(2) Holographic reflecting areas:

The holographic reflecting areas (Fig. 2-19) on the dorsal side of hand are similar to those on the palmar side. These extraordinarily sensitive areas should be selected to apply stimulation for relieving sensitivity, even though there is no disease in their correspondent organs. Diagnosing diseases by means of the hand will be discussed in following chapters.

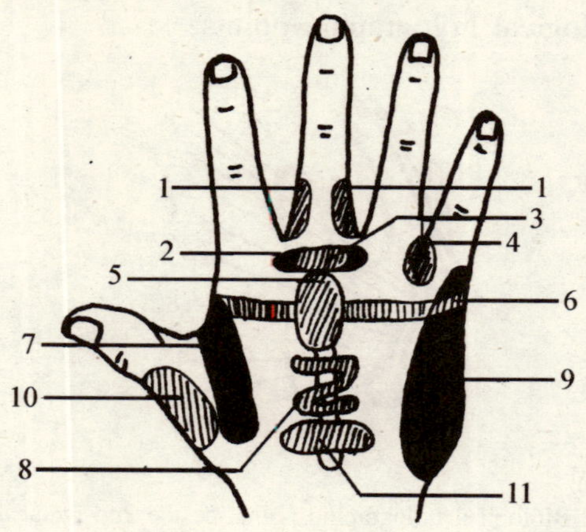

Fig. 2-19 Holographic reflecting areas on dorsum of hand

1-shoulder 2-neck 3-pharynx 4-ear 5-diaphragm 6-chest 7-nerve and blood pressure 8-abdomen 9-reflecting area of spine 10-endocrine 11-waist and leg

The anatomy of the hand and acupoints and reflecting areas for therapy applied to the hand have been mentioned above. Although the acupoints and reflecting areas are numerous, their names and locations can be gradually remembered by repeated recitation and clinical practice.

II. Anatomy, Acupoints and Reflecting Areas of Foot

1. Anatomy of the foot:

Following the differentiation of the hand and foot through human development, the feet bear the responsibility of supporting the body, and so the foot is, of course, far inferior to the hand in performing skillful movements. The anatomy of the foot, as that of the hand, has drawn the attention of scholarly investigation, although its responsibilities are simpler and less abstruse.

The feet are the lowest part of the body. When people stand and walk they must keep the body stable. For accomplishing their specific functions, the feet have a unique anatomic structure and a complicated blood supply and nervous system to regulate the body's repeated movements and constant change of posture. Mankind achieved the ability to stand up and walk on two feet through exercise over the millennia, as individuals obtain their ability to walk after exercise beginning in early childhood. Therefore, exercise was essential to the development of the foot, and remains so. The foot is the stablizing part of the body, just as the hand is the skillful member.

In normal people, the foot is composed of 26 bones. Among them are the 7 tarsal bones: the calcaneous, talus, cuboid, navicular and 1st, 2nd and 3rd cuneiform bones; they are connected by the articular ligaments to perform dorsiflexion, plantar flexion, and rotation of the ankle joint. The 5 metatarsal bones are arranged in a parallel pattern from the big toe to the

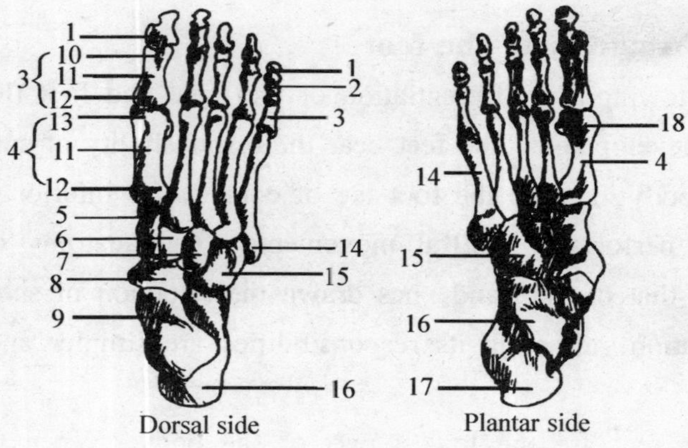

Fig. 2-20 Bones of foot

1-distal phalanx 2-middle phalanx 3-proximal phalanx 4-1st metacarpal bone 5-1st cuneiform bone 6-2nd cuneiform bone 7-3rd cuneiform bone 8-navicular bone 9-talus bone 10-trochlea 11-body 12-base 13-caput 14-5th metatarsal bone 15-cuboid bone 16-calcaneous bone 17-calcaneous tuberosity 18-sesamoid bone.

little toe and are numbered from 1st to 5th. The toes contain 14 phalanges, 2 in the big toe and 3 in each of other toes, and they are numbered as 1st (proximal), 2nd (middle) and 3rd (distal) phalanx from the proximal end to distal end of a toe. The bones of the foot are connected by muscles, tendons, and fibrous bundles to perform different foot movements. (Fig. 2-20).

There are also numerous blood vessels (Fig. 2-21) and

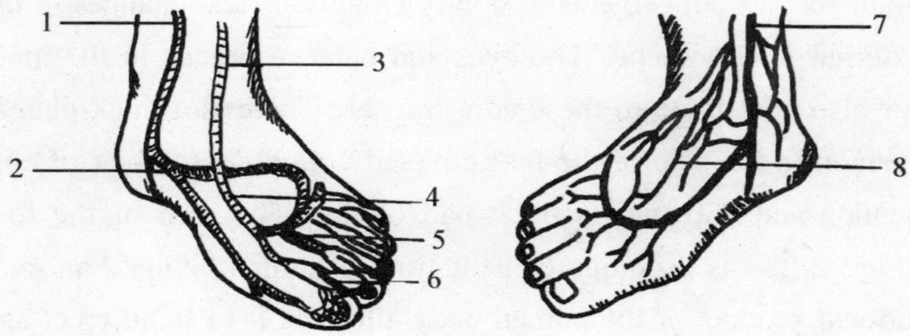

Fig. 2-21 Distribution of blood vessels in foot

1-posterior tibial artery 2-plantar artery 3-anterior tibial artery 4-dorsal foot artery 5-arcuate artery 6-dorsal metatarsal artery 7-anterior tibial vein 8-dorsal venous rete of foot

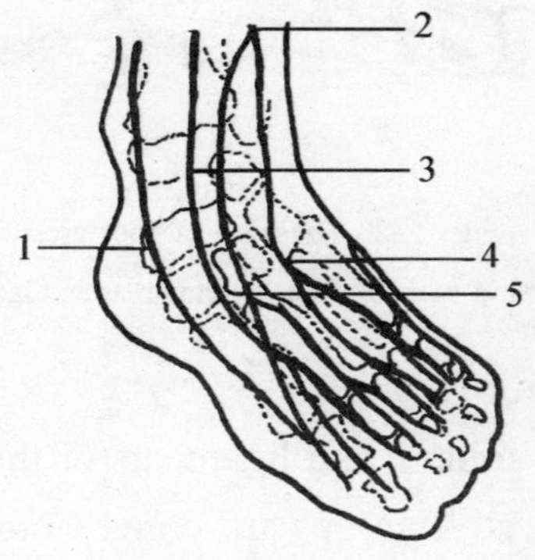

Fig. 2-22 Distribution of nerves in foot

1-saphenous nerve 2-superficial peroneal nerve 3-deep peroneal nerve 4-lateral dorsal cutaneous foot nerve 5-intermediate dorsal cutaneous foot nerve

nerve branches with nerve endings and receptors distributed in the foot (Fig. 2-22) to conduct nerve impulses to and from the brain for fast adjustments to bodily conditions and changes in the external environment. The eyes and balance organs in the inner ear also contribute to these adjustments. There is a thick plantar cushion in the sole of the foot covered with a dense layer of epithelium and laid over a thick pad of fat. The arch of the foot (Fig. 2-23) is a unique construction in human beings, an evolutional product of the human body allowing it to stand erect and

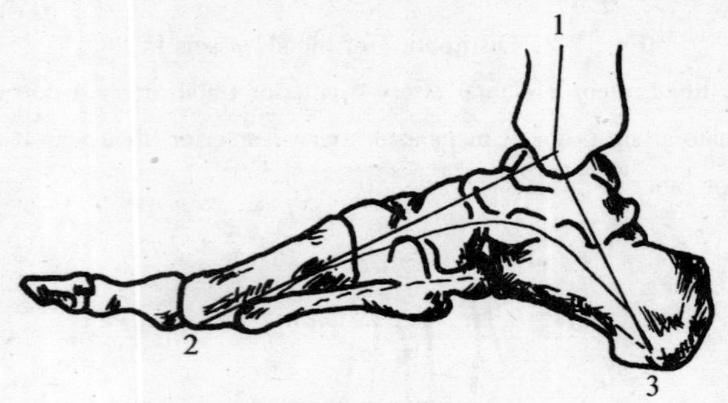

Fig. 2-23 Diagram of foot arch

1-gravity line 2-transverse arch of foot 3-plantar arch (lateral and medial longitudinal arches of foot)

walk. The bones, joints, and ligaments of the foot are arranged in a bow-like arch with an upward convex curvature to form the elastic structure of the arch. The rebound force from the ground when walking, jumping or bearing heavy weight is thereby diverted and reduced by the arch of the foot to protect the internal organs and tissues from injury. It also protects the nerves and blood vessels in the sole when standing or bearing weight for a long time. The arch consists of the longitudinal arch, anteroposteriorly arranged, and the transverse arch, mediolaterally arranged. To protect the arch of the foot, physical exercise is recommended to strengthen the foot muscles, ligaments and bones. Standing in a static posture over a long time should be avoided. Walking, running and jumping capability may be severely impaired in patients with flat feet.

The foot has been called a "second heart" or "third eye" of the human body because it can play a role in adjusting essential body organs such as the heart and eye through the close connection between the foot and the internal organs. As with the hand, the electrical activity of the foot is very similar to that of the head. The foot is sensitive to changes in temperature and can rapidly affect the functioning of the respiratory, circulatory, and digestive systems. There is a folk proverb: "The whole body feels warm if the foot is warm, and the whole body feels cool if the foot is cool." The aging process, bodily instability, and many diseases often start in the lower limbs. The head, hands and feet are similarly distant from the anatomical and gravitational center of the body. Therefore, an important function is particularly committed to these "periperal structures" of the body.

2. General principles of acupoints and reflecting areas on foot:

According to the meridian theory of traditional Chinese medicine, 6 regular meridians, including the foot Yangming stomach, foot Taiyang uninary bladder, foot Shaoyang gallbladder, foot Shaoyin kidney, foot Jueyin liver, and foot Taiyin spleen meridians are connected with the foot, and 33 regular acupoints having important therapeutic functions are located at the original or terminal parts of these 6 meridians.

Through continuous clinical practice, 74 extra foot acupoints were discovered and put into therapeutic use.

These holographic points and reflecting areas are widely distributed on the foot, produce stable therapeutic effects, and are not difficult to remember and use in clinical practice.

The acupoints and reflecting areas on the hand and foot can be used independently or in combination to produce an adjusting effect anywhere in the body depending on the time and place of treatment, the nature of the disease, and the experience of the practioner.

3. Distribution of acupoints and reflecting areas on plantar side of foot:

The plantar side of the foot has 1 regular acupoint, 43 extra acupoints, and 32 holographic points and reflecting areas as follows:

1) Regular acupoint:

Yongquan (KI 1):

Location: On the longitudinal midline and at the junction of anterior one-third and posterior two-thirds of the sole, at the tip of a V-shaped crease (Fig. 2-24).

Indications: Fainting, psychosis, convulsions, sore throat,
dryness in mouth, diarrhea, dryness and rhagades of foot, shock, hypertension, stroke, heat stroke, insomnia, heart palpitations, heart pain, vertigo, parietal headache, prolapse of uterus, infertility, aphonia, dysurination, constipation, and spasms due to cholera.

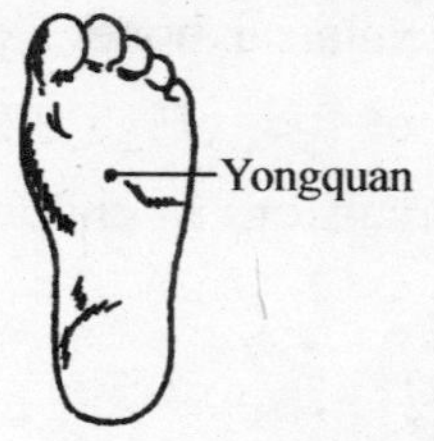

Fig. 2-24 Yongquan (KI 1) acupoint

2) Extra acupoints:

(1) Insomnia (Anmian) acupoint (EX-PF 1):

Location: At the center of the sole (Fig. 2-25).

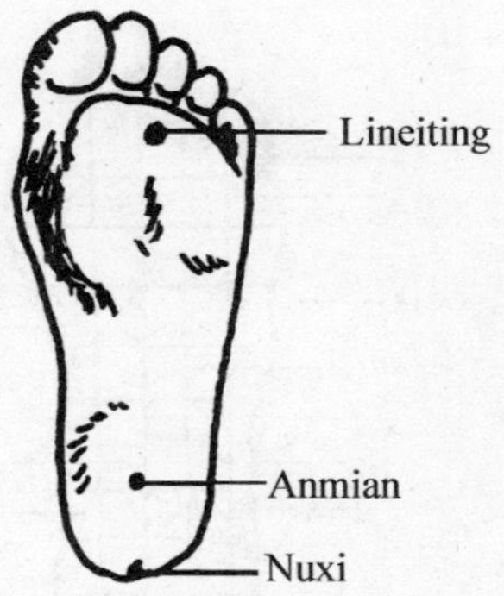

Fig. 2-25 Extra acupoints on plantar side of foot

Indication: Insomnia.

(2) Lineiting (inner Neiting) acupoint (EX-PF 2):

Location: On the plantar side of foot and in the interosseous space between 2nd and 3rd metatarsal bones, and opposite to Neiting (ST 44) on dorsal side of foot (Fig. 2-25).

Indications: Pain of toes, convulsions in children, indigestion, and epilepsy.

(3) Nuxi acupoint (EX-PF 3):

Location: At the midpoint of posterior heel border and on the dorsoplantar boundary of the foot (Fig. 2-25).

Indications: Alveolitis, alveolar abscess, convulsions, epilepsy, nasal bleeding, and nasal obstruction.

(4) No. 1 acupoint (EX-PF 4):

Location: This is 1 cun anterior to the midpoint of posterior heel border (Fig. 2-26).

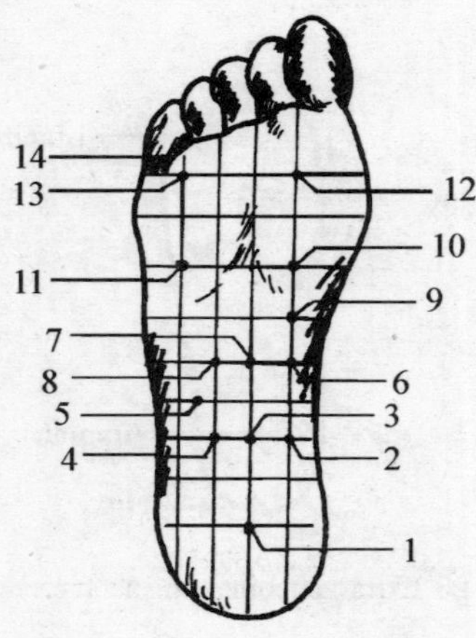

Fig. 2-26 No. 1 to No. 14 extra acupoints on plantar side of foot

Indications: Common cold, headache, maxillary sinusitis, and rhinitis.

(5) No. 2 acupoint (EX-PF 5):

Location: This is 3 cun anterior to the posterior heel border and 1 cun medial to the midline of sole (Fig. 2-26).

Indication: Trigeminal neuralgia.

(6) No. 3 acupoint (EX-PF 6):

Location: This is 3 cun anterior to the posterior heel border (Fig. 2-26).

Indications: Neurasthenia, hysteria, insomnia, hypotension, and coma.

(7) No. 4 acupoint (EX-PF 7):

Location: This is 3 cun anterior to the posterior heel border and 1 cun lateral to the midline of sole (Fig. 2-26).

Indications: Intercostal neuralgia, chest pain, and chest distress.

(8) No. 5 acupoint (EX-PF 8):

Location: This is 4 cun anterior to the posterior heel border and 1.5 cun lateral to the midline of sole (Fig. 2-26).

Indications: Sciatic neuralgia, appendicitis, and chest pain.

(9) No. 6 acupoint (EX-PF 9):

Location: This is 5 cun anterior to the posterior heel border and 1 cun medial to the midline of sole (Fig. 2-26).

Indications: Dysentery, diarrhea, and duodenal peptic ulcer.

(10) No. 7 acupoint (EX-PF 10):

Location: This is 5 cun anterior to the posterior heel border (Fig. 2-26).

Indications: Asthma and maldevelopment of brain.

(11) No. 8 acupoint (EX-PF 11):

Location: This is 1 cun lateral to No. 7 acupoint (Fig. 2-26).

Indications: Neurasthenia, epilepsy, and psychoneurosis.

(12) No. 9 acupoint (EX-PF 12):

Location: This is 4 cun posterior to the junction of big and second toes (Fig. 2-26).

Indications: Dysentery, diarrhea, and uteritis.

(13) No. 10 acupoint (EX-PF 13):

Location: This is 1 cun medial to Yongquan (KI 1) acupoint (Fig. 2-26).

Indications: Chronic gastroenteritis and stomach spasms.

(14) No. 11 acupoint (EX-PF 14):

Location: This is 2 cun lateral to Yongquan (KI 1) acupoint (Fig. 2-26).

Indications: Shoulder pain and urticaria.

(15) No. 12 acupoint (EX-PF 15):

Location: This is 1 cun posterior to the junction of big and second toes (Fig. 2-26).

Indication: Toothache.

(16) No. 13 acupoint (EX-PF 16):

Location: This is 1 cun posterior to the midpoint of plantar crease of little toe (Fig. 2-26).

Indication: Toothache.

(17) No. 14 acupoint (EX-PF 17):

Location: This is at the midpoint of plantar crease of little toe (Fig. 2-26).

Indications: Frequent urination and incontinence of urine.

Notice: The midline of the sole is a line between the junction of 2nd and 3rd toes and the midpoint of posterior heel border, and it is divided into 10 proportional cun of the patient's body. Three lines are drawn from each junction of 2 neighboring toes and parallel to the midline to a distance of 1 cun between each of the 2 neighboring lines. The horizontal lines are drawn to a distance of 1 cun between 2 neighboring lines to form a network. There are also other acupoints on this network.

(18) Regeneration acupoint (EX-PF 18):

Location: This is 5 fen posterior to No. 3 acupoint (Fig. 2-27).

Indications: Malignant brain tumors, nasal bleeding, and nasal obstruction.

(19) Eye acupoint (EX-PF 19):

Location: This is 5 fen anterior to No. 2 acupoint (Fig. 2-27).

Indications: Redness, swelling, and pain of eye.

(20) Head acupoint (EX-PF 20):

Location: This is 5 fen anterior to No. 3 acupoint (Fig. 2-27).

Indications: Headache and insomnia.

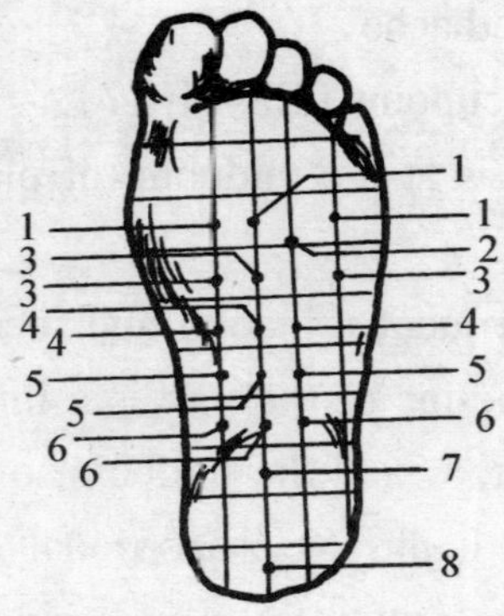

Fig. 2-27 Extra acupoints on plantar side of foot

1-liver, kidney and gallbladder 2-pain-controlling 3-lung, heart and urinary bladder 4-spleen, pericardium and triple energizer 5-colon, stomach and small intestine 6-eye, head and ear 7-regeneration 8-mouth

(21) Ear acupoint (EX-PF 21):

Location: This is 5 fen anterior to No. 4 acupoint (Fig. 2-27).

Indications: Nervousness and pain.

(22) Colon acupoint (EX-PF 22):

Location: This is 5 fen posterior to No. 6 acupoint and 1 cun anterior to eye acupoint (Fig. 2-27).

Indications: Abdominal pain, diarrhea, appendicitis, and acute stomachache.

(23) Stomach acupoint (EX-PF 23):

Location: This is 1 cun lateral to colon acupoint (Fig. 2-

27).

Indications: Psychosis, acute stomachache, abdominal pain, diarrhea, appendicitis, toothache, and osteomyelitis of maxillary bone.

(24) Small intestine acupoint (EX-PF 24):

Location: This is 1 cun lateral to stomach acupoint (Fig. 2-27).

Indications: Abdominal pain, diarrhea, appendicitis, and retention of urine.

(25) Spleen acupoint (EX-PF 25):

Location: This is 1 cun anterior to colon acupoint (Fig. 2-27).

Indications: Hernia with pain, testitis, convulsions in children, stroke with aphasia, acute stomachache, and emission of sperm.

(26) Pericardium acupoint (EX-PF 26):

Location: This is 1 cun anterior to stomach acupoint (Fig. 2-27).

Indications: Psychosis and insomnia.

(27) Triple energizer acupoint (EX-PF 27):

Location: This is 1 cun anterior to small intestine acupoint (Fig. 2-27).

Indications: Cough, chest pain, retention of urine, and tinnitus.

(28) Lung acupoint (EX-PF 28):

Location: This is 1 cun anterior to spleen acupoint (Fig.

2-27).

Indications: Cough and chest pain.

(29) Heart acupoint (EX-PF 29):

Location: This is 1 cun anterior to pericardium acupoint (Fig. 2-27).

Indications: Hypertension, psychosis, high fever with coma, stroke with aphasia, emission of sperm, and insomnia.

(30) Pain-controlling acupoint (EX-PF 30):

Location: This is 1 cun medial to No. 11 acupoint (Fig. 2-27).

Indications: Lumbago, acute and chronic gastroenteritis, and dysmenorrhea.

(31) Urinary bladder acupoint (EX-PF 31):

Location: This is 5 fen posterior to No. 11 acupoint (Fig. 2-27).

Indications: Retention of urine, nasal bleeding, nasal obstruction, and tinnitus.

(32) Liver acupoint (EX-PF 32):

Location: This is 1 cun anterior to lung acupoint (Fig. 2-27).

Indications: Hernia with pain, testitis or pain of testis, hypertension, psychosis, high fever with coma, convulsions in children, stroke with aphasia, emission of sperm, headache, and redness, swelling and pain of eye.

(33) Kidney acupoint (EX-PF 33):

Location: This is 1 cun lateral to liver acupoint (Fig. 2-

27).

Indications: Hernia with pain, testitis, hypertension, high fever with coma, convulsions in children, stroke with aphasia, cough, pain in flank, retention of urine, emission of sperm, toothache, osteomyelitis of maxillary bone, headache, and redness, swelling and pain of eye.

(34) Gallbladder acupoint (EX-PF 34):

Location: This is 5 fen anterior to No. 11 acupoint (Fig. 2-27).

Indications: Hypertension, high fever with coma, convulsions in children, cough, pain in flank, and tinnitus.

(35) Three Ludi acupoints (EX-PF 35):

Location: These are on the plantar side of foot, and the middle acupoint is 1.5 cun anterior to the cross point of a connecting line of tips of both malleoli and midline of sole, and the other two acupoints are 5 fen from and beside the middle one (Fig. 2-28).

Indications: High fever, headache, tinnitus, stomachache, pain of spleen and liver, constipation, abdominal distension, enteritis, dysentery, ascites, edema, mastitis, and paralysis.

(36) Aigen 1 acupoint (EX-PF 36):

Location: On the plantar side of foot, at the 1st tarsometatarsal joint, one finger width medial to dorsoplantar boundary of foot and at the lateral border of flexor muscle of big toe (Fig. 2-28).

Indications: Cancer of esophagus, stomach, and liver;

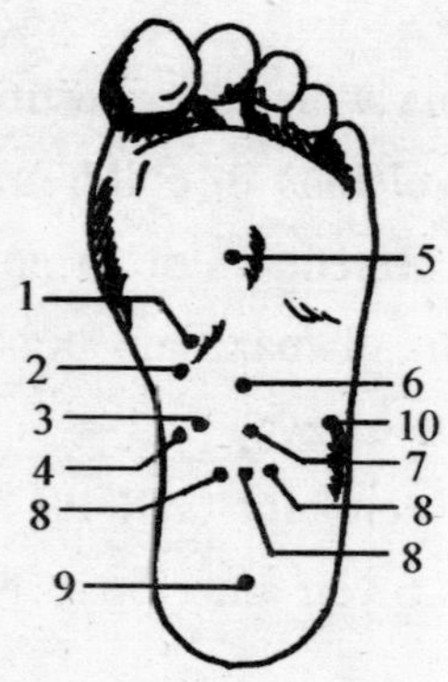

Fig. 2-28 Extra acupoints on plantar side of foot

1-Aigen 1 2-Aigen 2 3-Aigen 3 4-medial Ququan 5-Quanding 6-Quanzhong
7-Quangen 8-three Ludi 9-Sibai at heel 10-lateral Ququan.

metastatic cancer in lymph nodes, and chronic granulocytic leukemia.

(37) Aigen 2 acupoint (EX-PF 37):

Location: On the plantar side of foot, posterior to the tarsometatarsal joint of big toe and one finger width medial to dorsoplantar boundary of foot (Fig. 2-28).

Indications: Cancer of esophagus, rectum and cervix of uterus; and metastatic cancer of lymph nodes.

(38) Aigen 3 acupoint (EX-PF 38):

Location: On the plantar side of foot, at the talometatarsal joint and one finger width medial to dorsoplantar boundary (Fig. 2-28).

Indications: Cancer of liver, nasopharynx, and breast.

(39) Quangen acupoint (EX-PF 39):

Location: On the plantar side of foot, 1.5 cun posterior to the midpoint of a connecting line between the tip of 2nd toe and midpoint of posterior heel border (Fig. 2-28).

Indications: Mental diseases, hysteria, and leg spasms.

(40) Quanzhong acupoint (EX-PF 40):

Location: On the plantar side of foot, 1 cun anterior to Quangen acupoint (EX-PF 39) along the line connecting tip of 2nd toe and midpoint of posterior heel border (Fig. 2-28).

Indications: Mental diseases, hysteria, leg spasms, and mania.

(41) Quanding acupoint (EX-PF 41):

Location: On the plantar side of foot, 1 cun anterior to the junction of anterior two-fifths and posterior three-fifths of a line connecting the tip of 2nd toe and midpoint of posterior heel border (Fig. 2-28).

Indications: Hysteria, mental diseases, leg spasms, and mania.

(42) Sibai acupoint at heel (EX-PF 42):

Location: On the plantar side of foot, at the junction of the midline of sole and a line drawn from the midpoint of a connecting line between the tip of lateral malleolus and heel tendon (Fig. 2-28).

Indications: Prolapse of anus, bed-wetting, headache, convulsions in children, hemiplegia, cerebrospinal meningitis, foot drop, and regurgitation of milk in babies.

(43) Medial and lateral Ququan acupoints (EX-PF 43):

Location: They are on the plantar side of foot. A horizontal line is drawn 3 cun anterior to Sibai acupoint at heel (EX-PF 42), the junction of this line with medial bordor of sole is the medial Ququan acupoint, and the junction of this line with lateral border of sole is the lateral Ququan acupoint (Fig. 2-28).

Indications: Talipes valgus, talipes varus, and paralysis of legs.

3) Holographic points and reflecting areas:

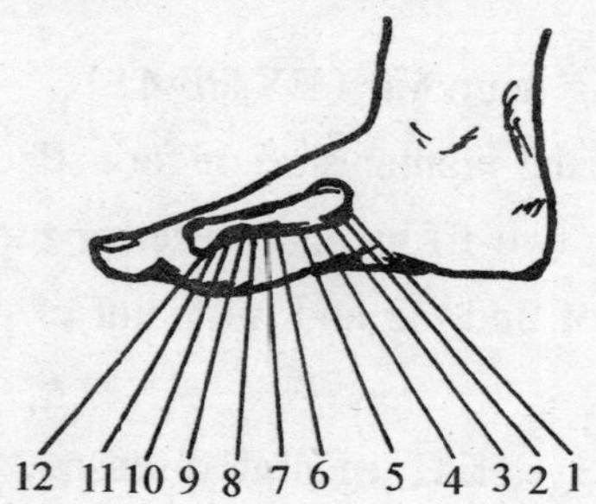

Fig. 2-29 Holographic points on plantar side of foot

1-head 2-neck 3-arm 4-lung and heart 5-liver 6-stomach 7-duodenum 8-kidney 9-waist 10-lower abdomen 11-leg 12-foot.

(1) Biological holographic points:

The arrangement of holographic points on the sole is similar to those on the hand, and the holographic points on the 1st metatarsal bone are commonly used in clinical practice. The holographic points between the 1st and 2nd metatarsal bones are more sensitive and may be selected for use according to the disease and the condition of the patient. (Fig. 2-29).

(2) Holographic reflecting areas:

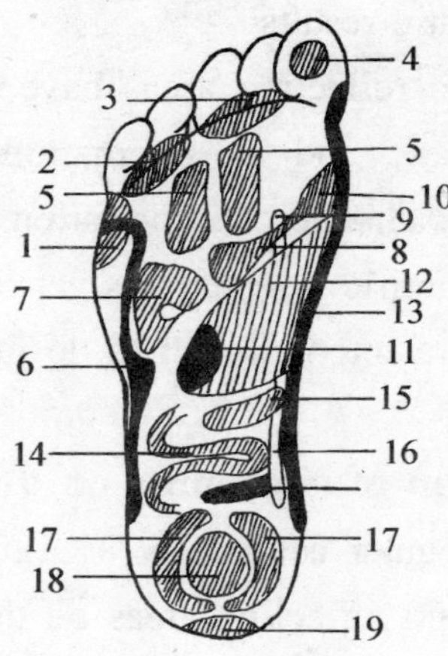

Fig. 2-30 Holographic reflecting areas on plantar side of foot

1-shoulder 2-ear 3-eye 4-brain 5-lung 6-lymphatic system (upper body to lower body) 7-liver and gallbladder 8-chest 9-cancer 10-heart 11-kidney 12-stomach 13-spinal column (cervical to lumbar and sacral region) 14-intestine 15-pancreas 16-urinary bladder 17-face 18-reproduction 19-anus

The holographic reflecting areas (Fig. 2-30) are the most important locations for applying massage therapy. They may be used as the principal location of treatment in combination with other acupoints or used independently. The maps of holographic reflecting areas drawn by different physicians vary, although most of them produce similarly good therapeutic results. Beginners may obtain good therapeutic results if they select one of the better holographic maps, but of course qualified physicians with rich knowledge and clinical experience will in any case be able to correctly select the holographic reflecting areas and produce much better therapeutic results.

The holographic reflecting areas have drawn the attention of many investigators, and an international organization has been set up for the exchange of information and experience, although profound scientific research has yet to be carried out and still awaits scholars talented enough to do just that.

4. Distribution of acupoints on dorsal side of foot:

There are 32 regular acupoints, 31 extra acupoints and 19 holographic points and reflecting areas on the dorsal side of the foot.

1) Regular acupoints:

(1) Rangu (KI 2):

Location: In a depression on the anteroinferior border of navicular bone (Fig. 2-31).

Indications: Irregular menstruation, hemoptysis, emission of sperm, prolapse of uterus, tetanus in newborn babies, diabetes mellitus, swelling in dorsum of foot, diseases of throat, heart and lungs, lockjaw, and tetanus.

(2) Taixi (KI 3):

Location: In a depression between medial malleolus and heel tendon (Fig. 2-31).

Indications: Toothache, tinnitus, diabetes mellitus, sore throat, hemoptysis, irregular menstruation, lumbago, frequent urination, insomnia, asthma, angina pectoris, emission of sperm, impotence, nephritis, alopecia, and cystitis.

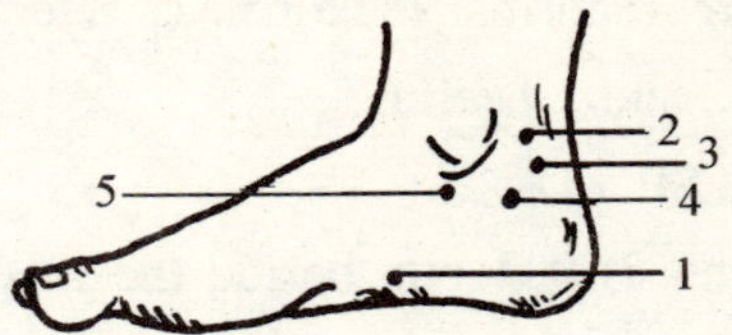

Fig. 2-31 Acupoints on kidney meridian on foot

1-Rangu (KI 2) 2-Taixi (KI 3) 3-Dazhong (KI 4) 4-Shuiquan (KI 5)
5-Zhaohai (KI 6)

(3) Dazhong (KI 4):

Location: This is 0.5 cun below and slightly posterior to Taixi (KI 3) and on the anterior border of heel tendon (Fig. 2-31).

Indications: Difficult urination, constipation, heel pain, dementia, hemoptysis, shortness of breath, toothache, stranguria, spasms of uterus, and lumbar neuralgia.

(4) Shuiquan (KI 5):

Location: In a depression on the anterior upper part of medial surface of calcaneal tuberosity and 1 cun directly below Taixi (KI 3) (Fig. 2-31).

Indications: Myopia, irregular menstruation, prolapse of uterus, and difficult urination.

(5) Zhaohai (KI 6):

Location: In a depression below the lower border of medial malleolus (Fig. 2-31).

Indications: Dryness in throat, irregular menstruation, prolapse of uterus, abnormal leukorrhea, retention of urine, insomnia, epilepsy, and hysteria.

(6) Yinbai (SP 1):

Location: This is 0.1 cun beside the medial corner of nail of big toe (Fig. 2-32).

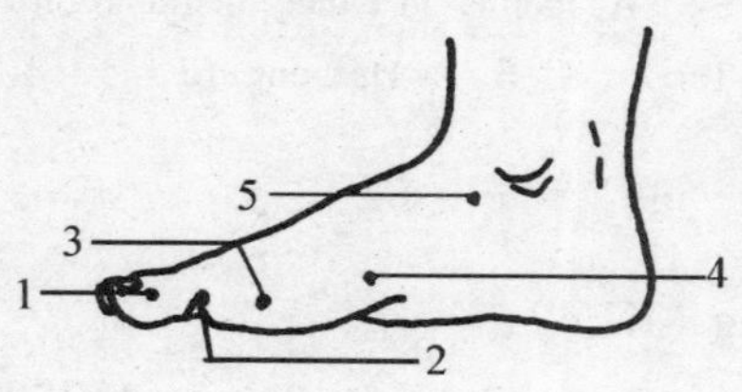

Fig. 2-32 Acupoints on spleen meridian on foot

1-Yinbai (SP 1) 2-Dadu (SP 2) 3-Taibai (SP 3) 4-Gongsun (SP 4) 5-Shangqiu (SP 5)

Indications: Abdominal distension, profuse menstrual discharge, psychosis, acute enteritis, digestive tract bleeding, chronic convulsions, and insomnia with many dreams.

(7) Dadu (SP 2):

Location: On the medial side of big toe, on the anterior border of 1st metacarpophalangeal joint and on the dorsoplantar boundary of the foot (Fig. 2-32).

Indications: Abdominal distension, stomachache, vomiting, diarrhea, febrile diseases without sweating, heaviness of body, pain in bones, irritability, convulsions in children, and cold limbs.

(8) Taibai (SP 3):

Location: On the posterior border of the capitulum of 1st metatarsal bone and on the dorsoplantar boundary of the foot (Fig. 2-32).

Indications: Abdominal distension, stomachache, vomiting, diarrhea, heaviness of body, indigestion of food, distension of chest and flank, increased abdominal gurgling, dysentery, constipation, neuralgia and paralysis of lower limbs, and soreness and pains in waist and thigh.

(9) Gongsun (SP 4):

Location: On the anterior border of base of 1st metatarsal bone and on the dorsoplantar boundary of the foot (Fig. 2-32).

Indications: Stomachache, vomiting, indigestion, abdominal pain, diarrhea, dysentery, epilepsy, and various urogenital diseases.

(10) Shangqiu (SP 5):

Location: In a depression 5 fen anterior to and below medial malleolus (Fig. 2-32).

Indications: Increased intestinal gurgling, abdominal distension, diarrhea, jaundice, indigestion, pain in foot and ankle, convulsions in children, hysteria, and stiff tongue.

(11) Dadun (LR 1):

Location: This is 0.1 cun beside the lateral corner of nail

ess, swelling and pain in eye, ... lapse of uterus, incontinence of ... nd constipation.

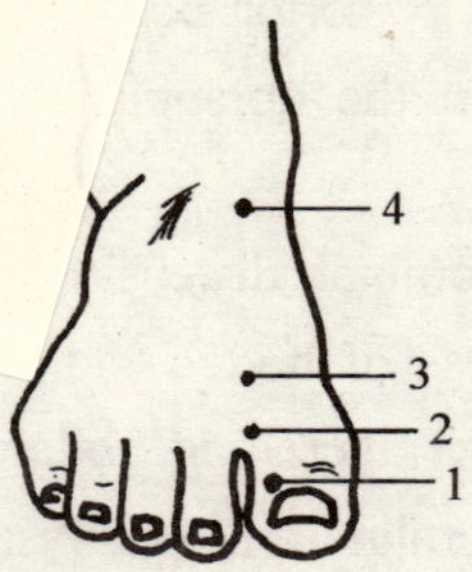

Fig. 2-33 Acupoints on liver meridian on foot

1-Dadun (LR 1) 2-Xingjian (LR 2) 3-Taichong (LR 3) 4-Zhongfeng (LR 4)

(12) Xingjian (LR 2):

Location: At the tip of a crease between 1st and 2nd meta-tarsophalangeal joints (Fig. 2-33).

Indications: Parietal headache, pain in flank, hernia with pain, night blindness, deviation of mouth, epilepsy, irregular menstruation, pain in urethra, incontinence of urine, difficult urination, constipation, hernia, irritability due to fever, insomnia, and knee joint pain.

(13) Taichong (LR 3):

Location: In a depression anterior to the junction of 1st and 2nd metatarsal bones (Fig. 2-33).

Indications: Diseases of liver and gallbladder, hypertension, hernia, profuse uterine bleeding, epilepsy, insomnia, vertigo, parietal headache, red eye, deviation of mouth, pain in flank, convulsions in children, difficult urination, and thrombocytopenia.

(14) Zhongfeng (LR 4):

Location: This is 1 cun anterior to medial malleolus and on the medial border of anterior tibial muscle (Fig. 2-33).

Indications: Hernia with pain, emission of sperm, anuresis, pain in penis, hepatitis, and ankle joint pain.

(15) Jiexi (ST 41):

Location: At the midpoint of dorsal crease of ankle joint and between the tendons of long extensor muscle of big toe and long extensor muscle of other toes (Fig. 2-34).

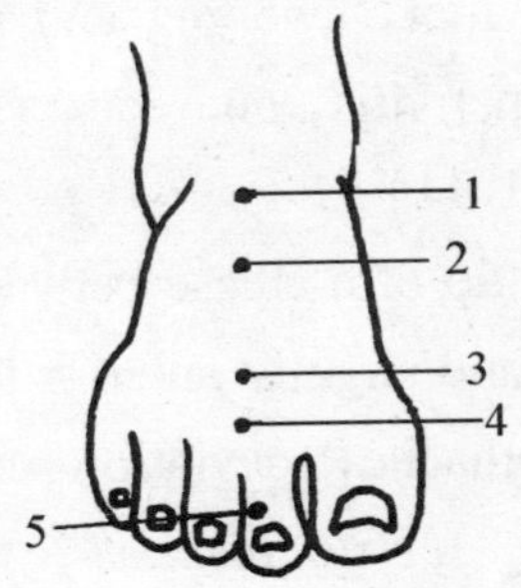

Fig. 2-34 Acupoints on stomach meridian on foot

1-Jiexi (ST 41) 2-Chongyang (ST 42) 3-Xian'gu (ST 43) 4-Neiting (ST 44)

5-Lidui (ST 45)

Indications: Headache, epilepsy, leg paralysis and pain, pain in ankle joint, indigestion, frontal headache, vertigo, abdominal distension with gas, enteritis, constipation, edema, and nephritis.

(16) Chongyang (ST 42):

Location: On the dome of foot dorsum in the interosseous space and 1.5 cun behind Jiexi (ST 41) (Fig. 2-34).

Indications: Deviation of mouth and eye, toothache, poor appetite, vomiting, trigeminal neuralgia, facial palsy, hardness and distension of abdomen, swelling and pain of foot dorsum, and psychosis.

(17) Xian'gu (ST 43):

Location: In a depression anterior to the conjuction of 2nd and 3rd metatarsal bones (Fig. 2-34).

Indications: Increase of intestinal gurgling, abdominal pain, pain in leg and foot, swelling and pain in foot dorsum, facial swelling, conjunctivitis, and edema.

(18) Neiting (ST 44):

Location: At the tip of a crease between 2nd and 3rd metatarsophalangeal joints and slightly anterior to them (Fig. 2-34).

Indications: Toothache, deviation of mouth, abdominal distension, dysentery, febrile diseases, trigeminal neuralgia, sore throat, nasal bleeding, stomachache, diarrhea, indigestion, pain in tarsal joints, foot swelling and pain, and hernia with pain.

(19) Lidui (ST 45):

Location: This is 0.1 cun beside the lateral corner of nail of 2nd toe (Fig. 2-34).

Indications: Pain in heart and abdomen, epilepsy, schizophrenia, sore throat, gingivitis, insomnia with many dreams, facial swelling, facial palsy, febrile diseases, and nasal bleeding.

(20) Qiuxu (GB 40):

Location: In a depression at the anteroinferior side of lateral malleolus and lateral to long extensor muscle of toes (Fig. 2-35).

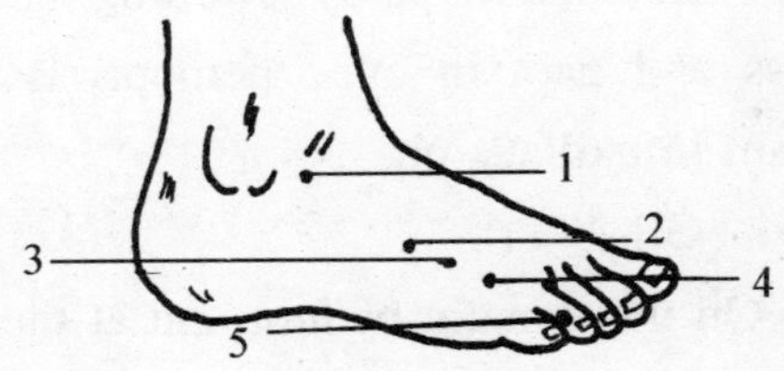

Fig. 2-35 Acupoints on gallbladder meridian on foot
1-Qiuxu (GB 40) 2-Zulinqi (GB 41) 3-Diwuhui (GB 42) 4-Xiaxi (GB 43)
5-Zuqiaoyin (GB 44)

Indications: Biliary colic, migraine, stiff neck, pain in chest and flank, malaria, leg paralysis, sciatic neuralgia, beriberi, hernia with pain, pain in neck and nape, and swelling and pain in ankle joint.

(21) Zulinqi (GB 41):

Location: In a depression anterior to the junction of 4th and 5th metatarsal bones and lateral to extensor muscle of little toe (Fig. 2-35).

Indications: Eye diseases, deafness, migraine, pain in chest and flank, biliary tract diseases, malaria, foot paralysis, foot spasms and pain, redness and swelling over tarsal bones, mastitis and tuberculosis of cervical lymph nodes.

(22) Diwuhui (GB 42):

Location: At the anterior part of foot dorsum, in a depression posterior to the junction of 4th and 5th tarsometatarsal joints (Fig. 2-35).

Indications: Rheumatic pain, swelling and pain in foot dorsum, redness and pain in eye, hemoptysis, mastitis, and swelling and pain in axillary pit.

(23) Xiaxi (GB 43):

Location: On the dorsum of foot and at the tip of a crease between 4th and 5th toes (Fig. 2-35).

Indications: Eye diseases, tinnitus, deafness, swelling of cheek, pain in chest and flank, febrile diseases, swelling and pain in foot dorsum, toe spasms, headache, edema of limbs, general body pain without fixed location, leg paralysis, hypertension, and hotness in sole of foot.

(24) Zuqiaoyin (GB 44):

Location: This is 0.1 cun beside the lateral corner of nail of 4th toe (Fig. 2-35).

Indications: Migraine, eye pain, pain in flank, febrile diseases, hiccups, cough with dyspnea, tinnitus, and dreaminess.

(25) Kunlun (BL 60):

Location: In a depression between lateral malleolus and

heel tendon（Fig. 2-36）:

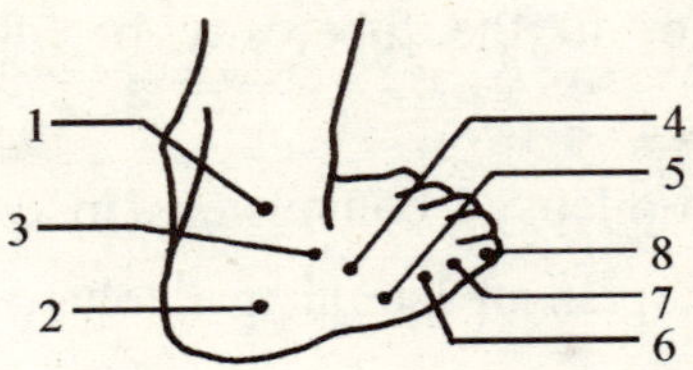

Fig. 2-36 Acupoints on urinary bladder meridian on foot
1-Kunlun（BL 60）2-Pucan（BL 61）3-Shenmai（BL 62）4-Jinmen（BL 63）
5-Jinggu（BL 64）6-Shugu（BL 65）7-Tonggu（BL 66）8-Zhiyin（BL 67）

Indications: Headache, stiff neck, pain in back and waist, pain in leg, heel swelling and pain, convulsions in children, epilepsy, prolonged labor, retention of placenta, vertigo, enlarged thyroid gland, nasal bleeding, and shoulder and arm spasms.

(26) Pucan（BL 61）:

Location: This is 1.5 cun below Kunlun（BL 60）（Fig. 2-36）.

Indications: Heel pain, foot paralysis, swelling and pain in knee joint, beriberi, epilepsy, and psychosis.

(27) Shenmai（BL 62）:

Location: In a depression at the lower border of lateral malleolus（Fig. 2-36）.

Indications: Headache, vertigo, sore pain in waist and leg, epilepsy, stroke, meningitis, and beriberi.

(28) Jinmen（BL 63）:

Location: On the lateral border of foot and in a depression above and posterior to the tuberosity of 5th metatarsal bone (Fig. 2-36).

Indications: Epilepsy, convulsions in children, deafness, tinnitus, lumbago, pain of lateral malleolus, frontal headache, and toothache.

(29) Jinggu (BL 64):

Location: On the dorsoplantar boundary below the tuberosity of 5th metatarsal bone (Fig. 2-36).

Indications: Headache, stiff neck, epilepsy, pain in waist and leg, myocarditis, meningitis, blurred vision, pain in knee joint, foot spasms, and nasal bleeding.

(30) Shugu (BL 65):

Location: On the lateral border of foot and in a depression above and posterior to 5th metatarsophalangeal joint (Fig. 2-36).

Indications: Epilepsy, dizziness, headache, eye diseases, fever, deafness, stiff neck, pain in lumbar and hip region, severe calf muscle pain, dysentery, and hemorrhoids.

(31) Tonggu (BL 66):

Location: On the lateral border of foot and in a depression anterior to and below 5th metatarsophalangeal joint (Fig. 2-36).

Indications: Headache, vertigo, nasal bleeding, stiff neck, congestion of blood in uterus, and psychosis.

(32) Zhiyin (BL 67):

Location: This is 0.1 cun beside the lateral corner of nail of little toe (Fig. 2-36).

Indications: Headache, eye pain, abnormal position of fetus, difficult labor, retention of placenta, nasal obstruction and bleeding, stroke, and emission of sperm.

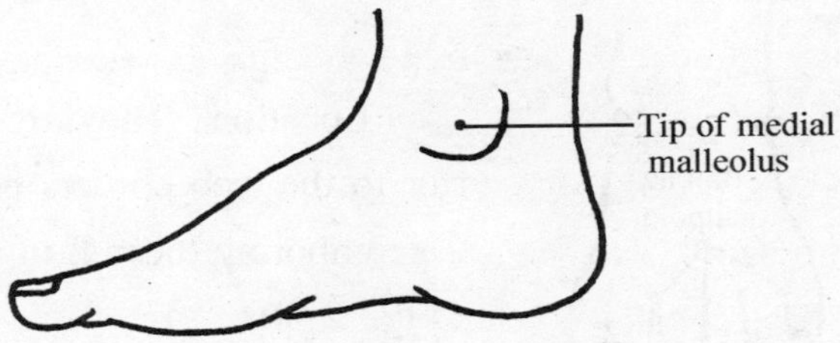

Fig. 2-37 Tip of medial malleolus acupoint

2) Extra acupoints:

(1) Tip of medial malleolus acupoint (EX-DF 1):

Location: At the tip of medial malleolus (Fig. 2-37):

Indications: Toothache of lower jaw, muscle spasms on medial side of foot, aphasia in babies and prolonged discharge of lochia.

(2) Tip of external malleolus acupoint (EX-DF 2):

Location: At the tip of lateral malleolus (Fig. 2-38).

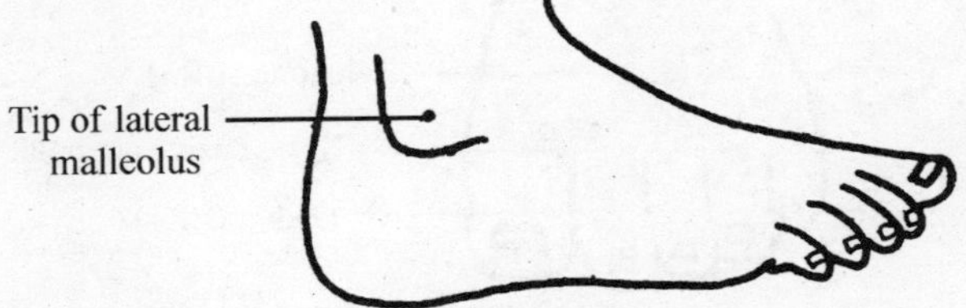

Fig. 2-38 Tip of lateral malleolus acupoint

Indications: Muscle spasms on the lateral side of foot, toe spasms, toothache, stranguria, inflammation of sublingual soft tissues in children, and beriberi.

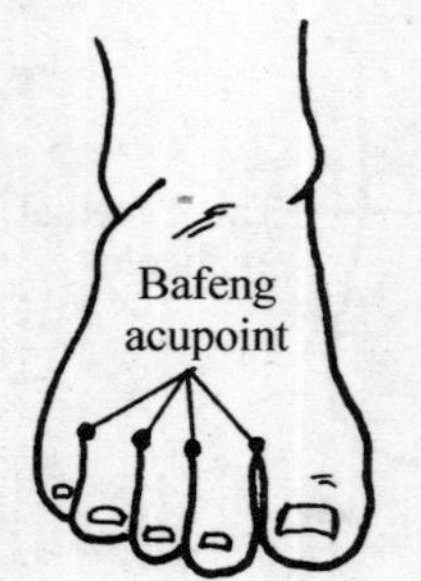

Fig. 2-39 Bafeng acupoint

(3) Bafeng acupoints (EX-DF 3):

Location: They are slightly posterior to the web borders between each of 2 neighboring toes, 8 in all on both feet (Fig. 2-39).

Indications: Redness and swelling of foot dorsum, beriberi, headache, neuralgia of dental nerves, intermittent fever, congestion of blood in lungs, irregular menstruation, malaria, and snake bite.

(4) Hypotensing acupoint (EX-DF 4):

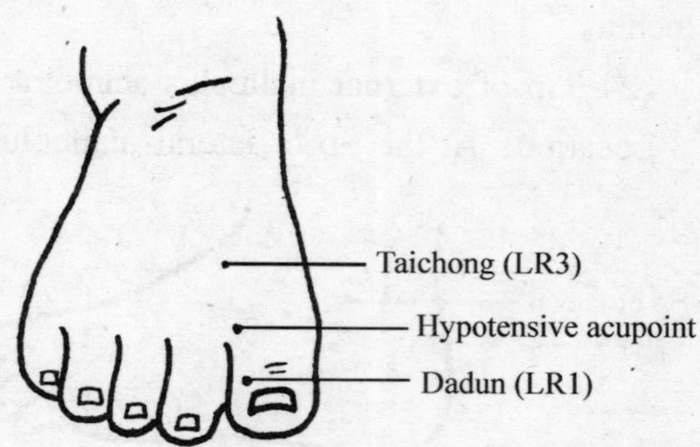

Fig. 2-40 Hypotensing acupoint

Location: On big toe and at the midpoint between Dadun (LR 1) and Taichong (LR 3) (Fig. 2-40).

Indication: Hypertension.

(5) Zhiping acupoints (EX-DF 5):

Location: They are on the dorsal side of toes and at the dorsal midpoints of each metatarsophalangeal joints, 10 in all on both feet (Fig. 2-41).

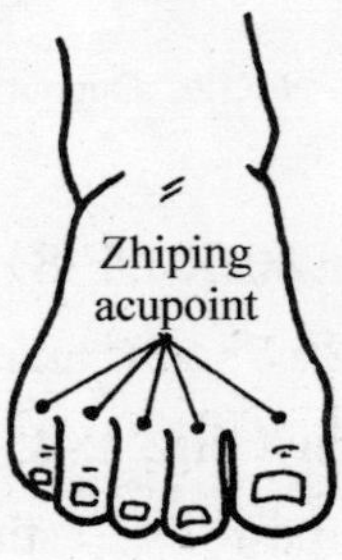

Fig. 2-41 Zhiping acupoints

Indications: Sequelae of poliomyelitis and paraplegia.

(6) No. 15 acupoints (EX-DF 6):

Location: These are 2 acupoints on each foot, 5 fen distal to the midpoint of dorsal crease of ankle joint and in the depressions (Fig. 2-42).

Indications: Pain in waist and leg and gastrocnemius muscle spasms.

(7) No. 16 acupoint (EX-DF 7):

Location: On the medial side of foot and in a depression above the process of navicular bone (Fig. 2-42).

Indications: Hypertension, parotitis, and acute tonsillitis.

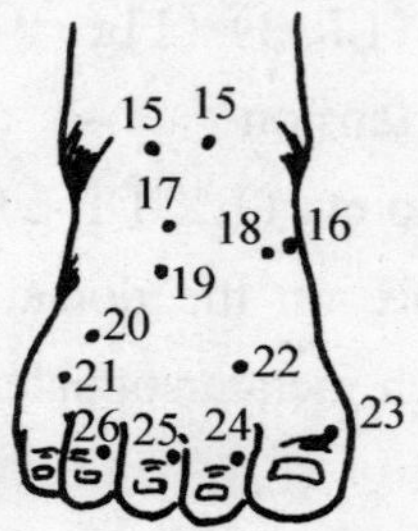

Fig. 2-42 No. 15 to No. 26 acupoints on dorsum of foot

(8) No. 17 acupoint (EX-DF 8):

Location: This is 2.5 cun anterior to the midpoint of dorsal crease of ankle joint (Fig. 2-42).

Indications: Angina pestoris, asthma, and common cold.

(9) No. 18 acupoint (EX-DF 9):

Location: In a depression anterior and medial to the caput of 1st metatarsal bone (Fig. 2-42).

Indications: Chest pain and distress, and acute waist sprain.

(10) No. 19 acupoint (EX-DF 10):

Location: This is 3 cun posterior to the junction of 2nd and 3rd toes (Fig. 2-42).

Indications: Headache, otitis media, acute and chronic gastroenteritis, and peptic ulcer of stomach and duodenum.

(11) No. 20 acupoint (EX-DF 11):

Location: This is 3 cum posterior to the junction of 3rd

and 4th toes (Fig. 2-42).

Indication: Stiff neck.

(12) No. 21 acupoint (EX-DF 12):

Location: This is 5 fen posterior to the junction of 4th and 5th toes (Fig. 2-42).

Indications: Sciatic neuralgia, parotitis, and tonsillitis.

(13) No. 22 acupoint (EX-DF 13):

Location: This is 1 cun posterior to the junction of 1st and 2nd toes (Fig. 2-42).

Indications: Acute tonsillitis, epidemic parotitis, and hypertension.

(14) No. 23 acupoint (EX-DF 14):

Location: On the metatarsophalangeal joint medial to the tendon of long extensor muscle of big toe (Fig. 2-42).

Indications: Acute tonsillitis, epidemic parotitis, hypertension, eczema, and urticaria.

(15) No. 24 acupoint (EX-DF 15):

Location: On the medial side of proximal interphalangeal joint of 2nd toe and on the dorsoplantar boundary (Fig. 2-42).

Indications: Headache and otitis media.

(16) No. 25 acupoint (EX-DF 16):

Location: On the medial side of proximal interphalangeal joint of 3rd toe and on the dorsoplantar boundary (Fig. 2-42).

Indication: Headache.

(17) No. 26 acupoint (EX-DF 17):

Location: On the medial side of proximal interphalangeal

joint of 4th toe and on the dorsoplantar boundary (Fig. 2-42).

Indications: Headache and hypotension.

(18) No. 27 acupoint (EX-DF 18):

Location: At the midpoint between Taibai (SP 3) and Gongsun (SP 4) acupoints (Fig. 2-43).

Indications: Epilepsy, hysteria, and abdominal pain.

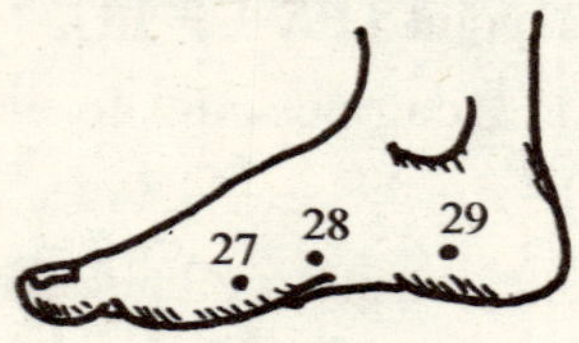

Fig. 2-43 No. 27 to No. 29 acupoints on medial side of foot

(19) No. 28 acupoint (EX-DF 19):

Location: On the medial side of foot and in a depression below and posterior to the process of navicular bone (Fig. 2-43).

Indications: Dysmenorrhea, functional uterine bleeding, and adnexitis.

(20) No. 29 acupoint (EX-DF 20):

Location: This 2 cun directly below the center of medial malleolus (Fig. 2-43).

Indications: Functional uterine bleeding, bronchitis, and asthma.

(21) No. 30 acupoint (EX-DF 21):

Location: This is 1.5 cun above and behind the lateral malleolus (Fig. 2-44).

Indications: Sciatic neuralgia, lumbago, and headache.

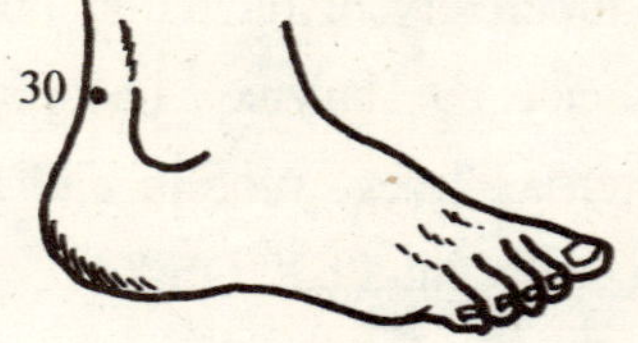

Fig. 2-44 No. 30 acupoint on foot

Notice: These numbered acupoints are located on the dorsum of foot according to the surface anatomy of the foot; the distance between the tips of medial and lateral malleoli and the lower border of medial and lateral sides of foot is divided into 3 cun.

(22) Chongshen acupoint (EX-DF 22):

Location: At a point of intersection between a vertical line 5 fen anterior to the medial malleolus and the dorsoplantar boundary (Fig. 2-45).

Indication: Inguinal hernia in children.

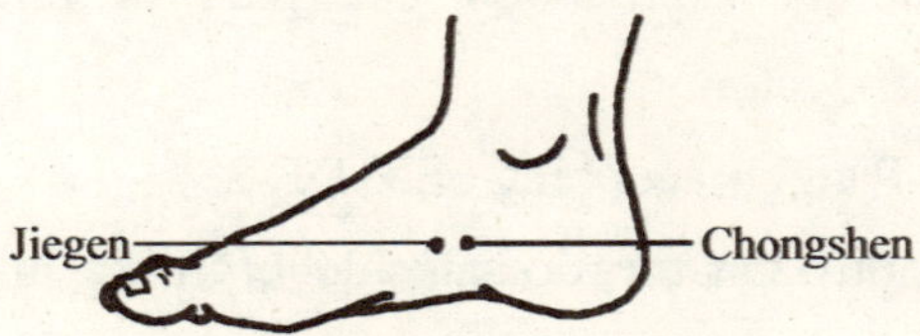

Fig. 2-45 Chongshen and Jiegen acupoints

(23) Jiegen acupoint (EX-DF 23):

Location: On the medial side of foot, 5 fen below a depression underneath the tuberosity of navicular bone (Fig. 2-45).

Indications: Cancer of larynx, nasopharynx, esophagus, stomach, breast, uterus, liver, rectum and lung.

(24) Relaxing acupoint (EX-DF 24):

Location: On the dorsum of foot, in a depression behind the posterior border of capitula of 2nd and 3rd metatarsal bones, but closer to the former bone (Fig. 2-46).

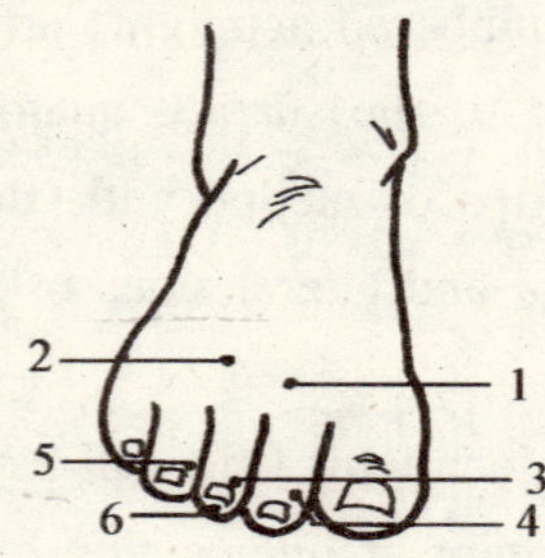

Fig. 2-46 Extra acupoints on dorsum of foot

1-relaxing 2-Panggu 3-Qingtou 1 4-Qingtou 2 5-Qingtou 3 6-Zuzhongchong.

Indication: Contraction and pain of abdominal muscles during appendectomy.

(25) Panggu acupoint (EX-DF 25):

Location: On the dorsal side of foot, at the junction between anteriorone-fourth and posterior three-fourths of the interosseous space between 3rd and 4th metatarsal bones (Fig. 2-46).

Indication: Sequelae of poliomyelitis.

(26) Qingtou 1 acupoint (EX-DF 26):

Location: On the dorsomedial border of distal interphalangeal joint of 2nd toe (Fig. 2-46).

Indications: Headache, common cold, neurasthenia, hysteria, acute otitis media, and lymphadenitis of lower jaw.

(27) Qingtou 2 acupoint (EX-DF 27):

Location: On the dorsomedial border of distal interphalangeal joint of 3rd toe (Fig. 2-46).

Indications: Headache and hypotension.

(28) Qingtou 3 acupoint (EX-DF 28):

Location: On the dorsomedial border of distal interphalangeal joint of 4th toe (Fig. 2-46).

Indications: Headache and neurasthenia.

(29) Zuzhongchong acupoint (EX-DF 29):

Location: At the tip of 3rd toe (Fig. 2-46).

Indications: Epilepsy, cardiac failure, and headache.

(30) Yejing acupoint (EX-DF 30):

Location: At the lateral end of distal interphalangeal crease of small toe (Fig. 2-47).

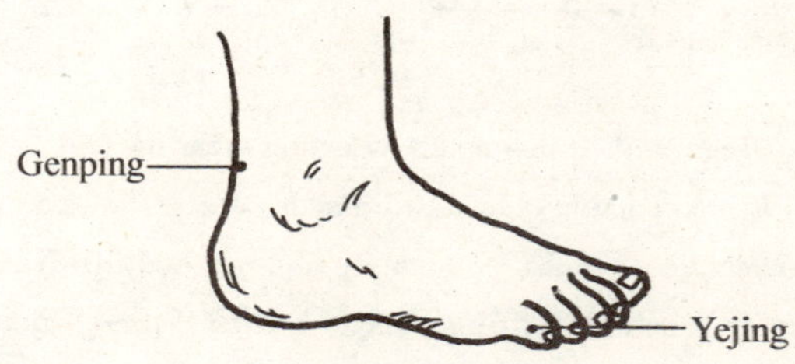

Fig. 2-47 Yejing and Genping acupoints

Indications: Bed-wetting, night blindness, and distension of eye.

(31) Genping acupoint (EX-DF 31):

Location: At the posterior midpoint of bilateral malleoli and on the tendon of triceps muscle of leg (Fig. 2-47).

Indications: Sequelae of poliomyelitis and foot drop.

3) Holographic points and reflecting areas:

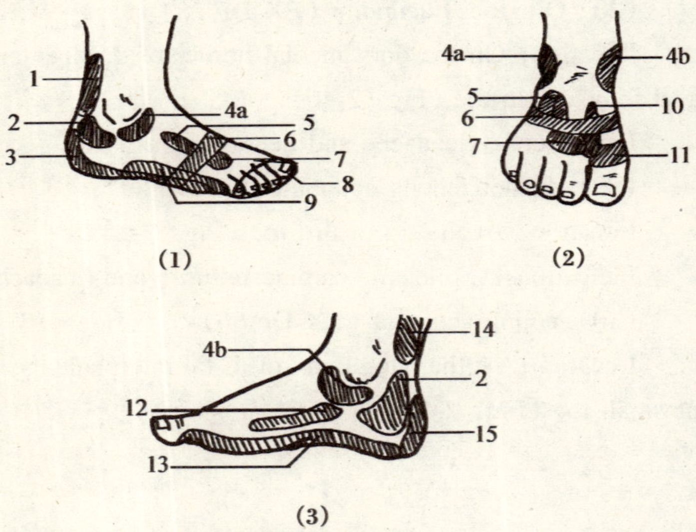

Fig. 2-48 Holographic reflecting areas on foot
1-pelvic cavity 2-reproductive organs and glands 3-muscular and skeletal region (coccyx to shoulder) 4a-lymphatic immunity of upper body 4b-lymphatic immunity of lower body 5-gallbladder 6-diaphragm 7-chest 8-head 9-immunity region 10-qi-stagnation zone 11-neck zone 12-abdominal distension 13-reflecting region of spinal column 14-rectum 15-anus areas.

92

The biological holographic points have been mentioned before; the holographic reflecting areas are also widely arrayed on the dorsum of foot (Fig. 2-48) and useful in clinical practice.

The holographic reflecting points and areas are a new development in acupuncture, brought about through the clinical experience of modern physicians, just as the application and accumulation of traditional acupoints was the invention and creation of traditional physicians over many centuries. If the acupoints on one side are projected on a map, most acupoints with similar locations and functions can be arranged in an area or a zone, although the acupoints and the projected areas are not completely correspondent. The application of holographic theory to medicine is not a new concept. The idea that there are correspondences between people and the universe, and that the human body is a miniature of the universe was expounded in ancient Chinese philosophy.

III. Therapeutic Mechanisms of Hand and Foot Massage

The massage at acupoints on both hand and foot can adjust bodily functions, promote the circulation of qi and blood, and prevent and treat diseases; and the effect of this therapy is even better than that of body massage and other local massages.

The therapeutic effects of hand and foot massage can be summarized into the following items for further investigation and scientific explanation.

1. Adjustment of nervous system:

As mentioned above, the electrical properties of the hand and foot is similar to those of the brain, but the reflex mechanisms of the nervous system are more complicated. Hand and foot massage can apply stimulation to the skin receptors and nerve endings of the hand and foot to adjust the internal organs after the stimulating impulse is transmitted through the vegetative nervous system. The stimulating impulse evoked by the massage to the terminal receptors (with some specificity) of the skin is first transmitted to the posterior horn of the spinal cord through afferent somatic nerve fibers; it is then conducted to the ventral posterolateral nucleus of the thalamus through the spinothalamic tract and projected to the postcentral gyrus through the occipital part of the internal capsule; the nerve impulse is again transmitted from the postcentral gyrus through efferent fibers to the reticular structure; and finally it is conducted to the internal organs through three routes. The first is from the reticular structure through the spinal nucleus of the vagus nerve, and parasympathetic fibers in vagus nerve to the internal organs; the second route is through the nucleus of the solitary tract, spinal nucleus of vagus nerve, and nerve fibers of vagus nerve to the internal organs; and the third route is from the reticular structure through the nucleus of the solitary tract to the center of sympathetic nervous system and then through the reticulospinal tract to the internal organs. As with other stimulation, the strong stimulation at short intervals can produce a stimulating effect; and the moderate stimulation at long intervals can produce an inhibitory effect. This phenomenon is a result of the adjustment between stimulation and inhibition by the cerebral cortex. During the application of hand and foot massage, the EEG may show a general exaggeration of alpha waves, even more apparent than that caused by other massage therapies.

2. Adjustment of blood and lymph system:

Hand and foot massage can promote circulation of the blood and lymphs, because its effect on local microcirculation quickly spreads to the entire body. As shown by experimental study, this massage can affect blood composition and the consumption of oxygen. The WBC count and ratio of lymphocytes in the blood were markedly increased; the neutrophils and RBC counts were also slightly increased. Oxygen consumption of the limbs can also be elevated to produce a general energetic metabolism keeping the body healthy through the adjustment of Ying (nutrients) and Wei (defensive energy) and promoting qi and blood circulation. After persistent stimulation applied to acupoints and reflecting areas of the hand and foot, the heart rate and breath frequence as well as oxygen consumption in patients undergoing operations can also be increased by this massage.

3. Adjustment similar to physical exercise:

It is well known that persistent and coordinated physical exercise can improve the adaptation, health and defensive energy of the body. Massage at a certain frequence, with certain pressure and over a certain period of time can adjust the functions of various internal organs and enhance the body's immune system. Although hand and foot massage is not a physical exercise done by the patient, it can produce similar effects as physical exercise. Why? The sum of the stimulating information available to the hand and foot through exercise is same as that produced by local massage applied to the hand and foot. Therefore, it produces a similar result. After strenuous mental activity over a long period of time, physical exercise can relieve mental fatigue. If the opportunity for physical exercise is not available, a self-massage on the hand and foot for a few minutes with eyes closed in an environment with fresh air can also achieve the same goal of mental refreshment.

4. Adjustment of meridian system:

As mentioned above, 12 important regular meridians originate from or stop at the hand or foot, and according to traditional medical theory they are closely related to the body's organs and tissues. The acupoints near the origin or terminal of meridians are more sensitive in the adjustment of meridians and the whole body, just as the water flowing in lower reaches is under the control of the water source from the upper reaches of a river. As proven in clinical practice, stimulation of the acupoints can produce a remarkable adjusting effect to the meridians and the entire body. Massage applied to the reflecting areas may unavoidably stimulate the acupoints in those areas. Once the mechanism of this adjusting effect can be scientifically illustrated, for example through a nerve-like channel, temporarily composed of cells, a new system—the meridian system of the body—can be proven and established on a scientific basis to explain the secrets of the human body.

5. Automatic adjustment of acupoints and reflecting areas on the hand and foot:

It has been proposed that there is an "adjusting chain" present in living organism as well as in non-living substances in the universe. This adjusting chain can also play its role in a small local portion of the body as well as in the entire body of a living organism. In brief, the acupoints on the hand are specifically related to their correlated organs, because they are all under the control of the adjusting chain. The stimulation applied at the acupoints and reflecting areas on the hand and foot can quickly and effectively adjust the function of their correlated organs and tissue.

6. Emphasis on massage at painful reactive areas:

Pain of the reactive areas is caused by the local accumulation of uric acid crystal, which is harmful to the body. Massage at this area can promote the discharge of uric acid, if enough water has been drunk, and can clear this toxic substance from the body to prevent and cure disease.

The foregoing discussion about the therapeutic mechanisms of hand and foot massage may help the reader understand the effects of this massage more profoundly, although final conclusion of these problems have not been settled yet. Therefore, the objective mechanism of hand and foot massage remain a puzzle waiting for an answer.

IV. Correlation Between Divisions of Hand and Foot and Internal Organs

For the convenience of learning and memory, the holographic acupoints and reflecting areas mentioned above are briefly summarized and shown in the following diagrams. However, these are only rough sketches and the exact location of stimulating areas must be accurately defined during clinical practice. As proven by clinical practice, good therapeutic results can be duplicated when similar stimulation is applied at the defined area.

1. Correspondent divisions of head and neck (Fig. 2-49a and Fig. 2-49b):

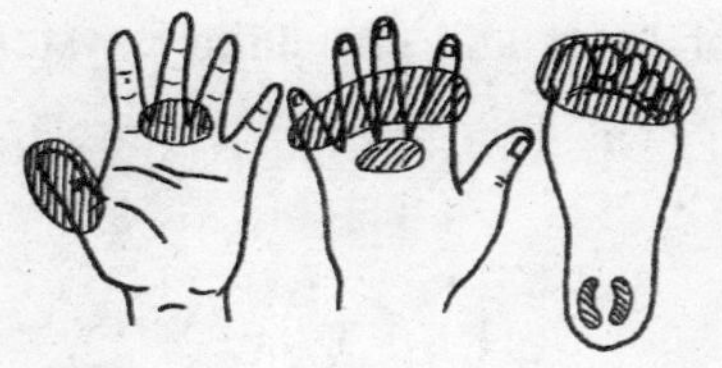
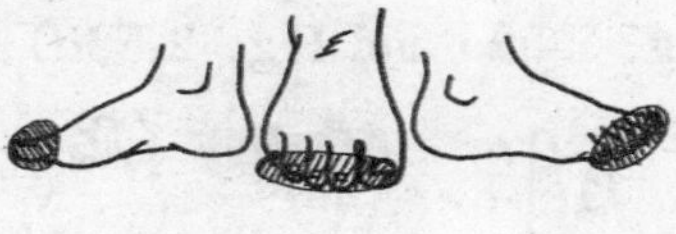

Fig. 2-49a   Fig. 2-49b

2. Correspondent divisions of lung and respiratory system (Fig. 2-50a and Fig. 2-50b):

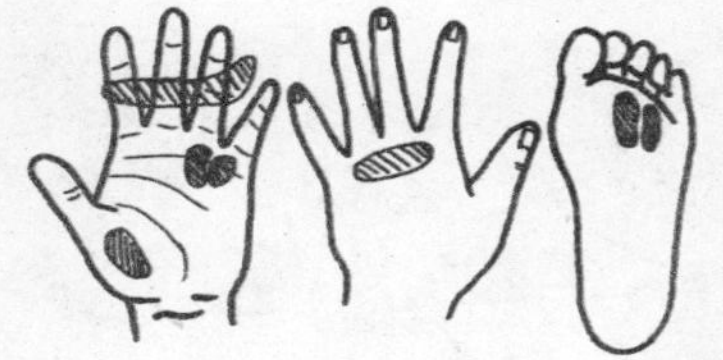
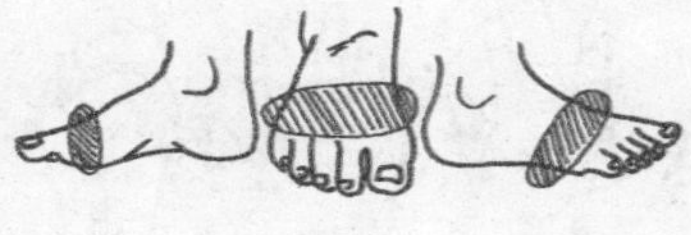

Fig. 2-50a   Fig. 2-50b

3. Correspondent divisions of spleen, stomach and digestive system (Fig. 2-51a and Fig. 2-51b):

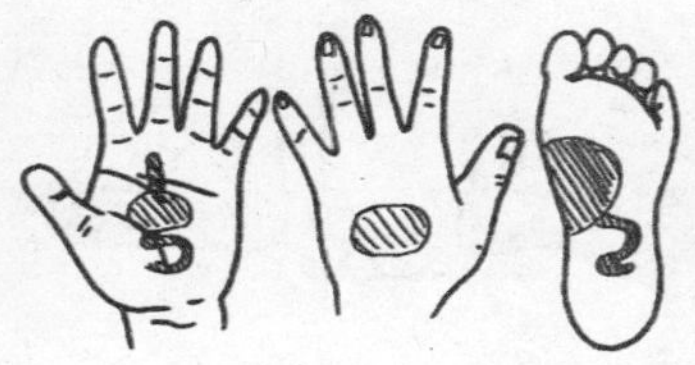
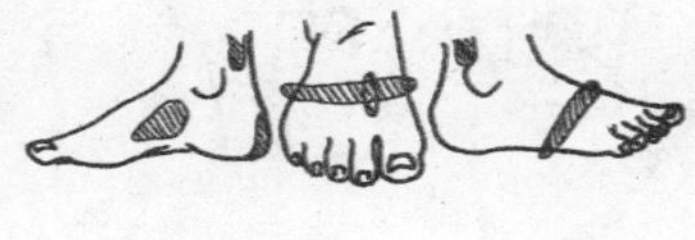

Fig. 2-51a   Fig. 2-51b

4. Correspondent divisions of heart and circulatory system (Fig. 2-52a and Fig. 2-52b):

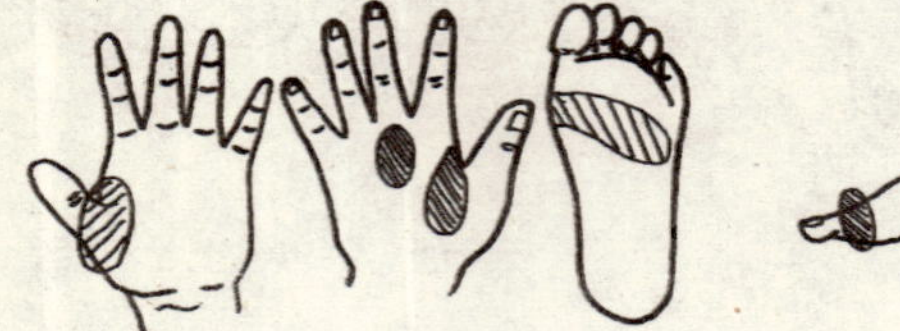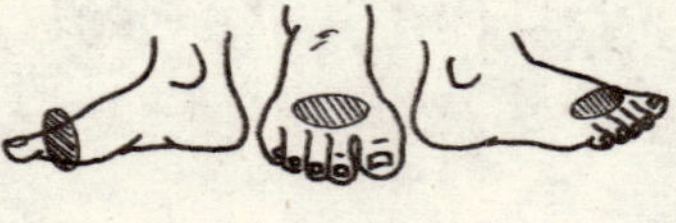

Fig. 2-52a   Fig. 2-52b

5. Correspondent divisions of kidney and urogenital system (Fig. 2-53a and Fig. 2-53b):

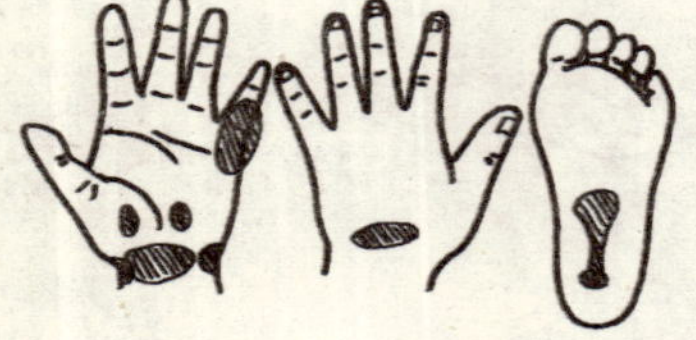

Fig. 2-53a   Fig. 2-53b

6. Correspondent divisions of brain and nervous system (Fig. 2-54a and Fig. 2-54b):

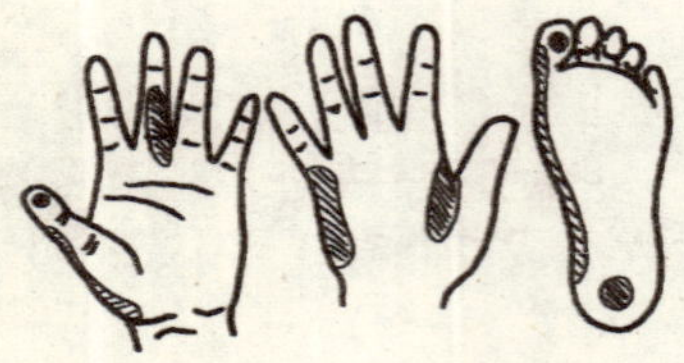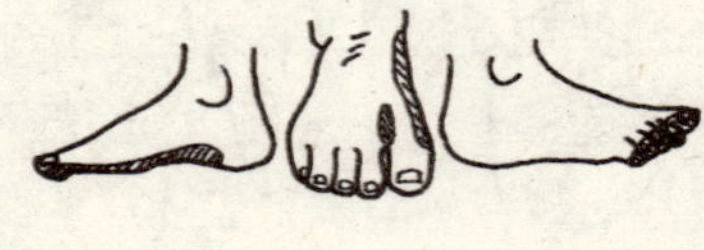

Fig. 2-54a   Fig. 2-54b

7. Correspondent divisions of endocrinal system (Fig. 2-55a and Fig. 2-55b):

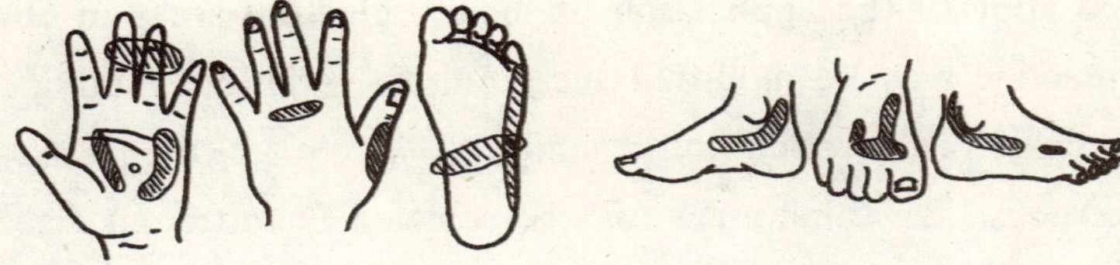

Fig. 2-55a   Fig. 2-55b

8. Correspondent divisions of lymphatic system (Fig. 2-56a and Fig. 2-56b):

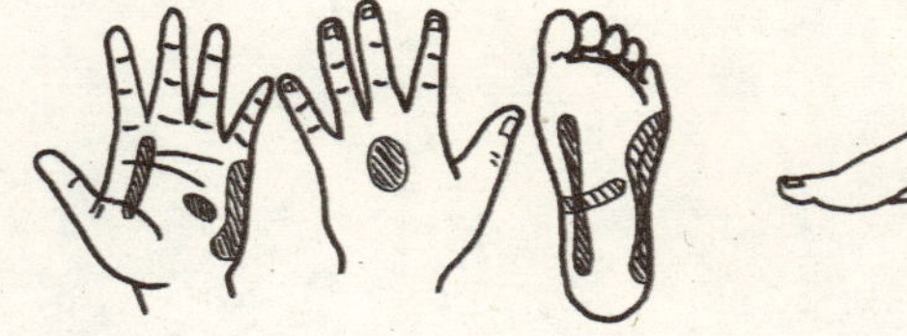

Fig. 2-56a   Fig. 2-56b

9. Correspondent divisions of locomotive system (Fig. 2-57a and Fig. 2-57b):

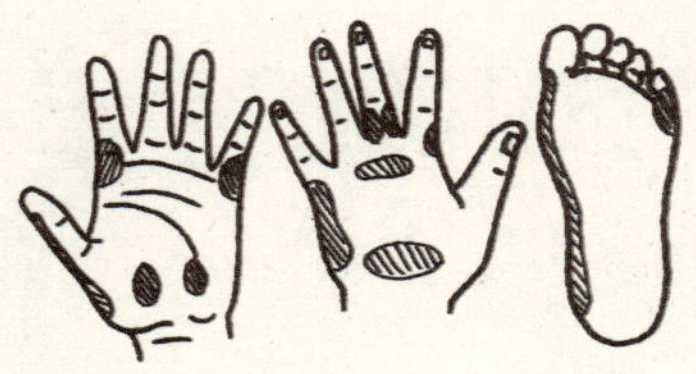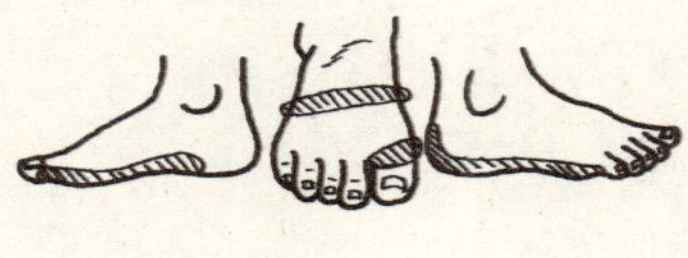

Fig. 2-57a   Fig. 2-57b

The vital organs and tissues in the body and their correspondent reflecting areas on the hand and foot have been mentioned above. The application of those reflecting areas in clinical practice may be modified according to variations among individuals, health conditions, and the nature of the disease. Sometimes, the same areas may be selected for different diseases; and similar diseases can be treated by different areas. These basic principles should be followed for smoothly solving the difficult problems that arise in the treatment of diseases.

CHAPTER 3 THERAPEUTIC MANEUVERS AND PRESCAUTIONS FOR MANIPULATION

I. General Discussion of Massage Maneuvers

A variety of skillful movements applied by the hand or other parts to specific acupoints and areas on the hand and foot are called massage maneuvers. Beginners may gradually learn and master these techniques by following the requirements or correct application and manipulation.

The basic requirements for successful application are persistence, forcefulness, evenness, and gentleness. Pressure should be applied deep enough to achieve the objective of functional adjustment. As persistence is essential, the maneuvers should be applied persistently for a period of time depending on therapeutic requirement. Manipulation with repeated intermissions and pauses cannot produce the proper effect. Therefore, beginners should constantly practice and do physical exercise to improve their force, skill, and persistence. The maneuvers should be applied with the right amount of force, otherwise the manipulation cannot produce the proper effect. At the same time, the force applied to the hand or foot should be modified according to the nature of the disease and the function of the acupoints and areas, because a fixed strong stimulation without correspondent modification may cause damage to the local tissue. The maneuvers should be evenly and rhythmically applied, with a stable frequency and coordinated force to producing a comfortable feeling and a sedative effect and securing the patient's cooperation. An irregular application of maneuvers with force and frequency changed in a disorderly manner from time to time may produce a bad feeling, annoy the patient, and reduce the therapeutic effect. Even application of maneuvers can be achieved after the beginner has learned how to persistently and forcefully apply them. The manipulation should be gentle, not violent, and changes should be smooth with the intensity of stimulation adequate for applying coordinated, continuous, and orderly massage. In brief, the techniques for persistently, forcibly, evenly, and gently applying maneuvers can be learned and mastered after careful trials and untiring practice.

The maneuvers usually applied in hand and foot massage including pressing, digit-pressing, pushing, pinching, twisting, rotating, pulling, rubbing, grinding and stepping maneuvers may be selected in accordance with the condition of patient and the nature of the disease.

1. Pressing maneuver:

Manipulation: The tip or pad of thumb (sometimes supported by another hand or applied by tip of elbow) is used to vertically apply pressure to the body surface. The finger should be firmly applied to the acupoint or area without any shift in location to avoid causing rubbing damage to the skin. The pressure should be gradually increased without any violent fluctuation. The frequency of vibration and the force applied to the acupoints or areas should be even (Fig. 3-1).

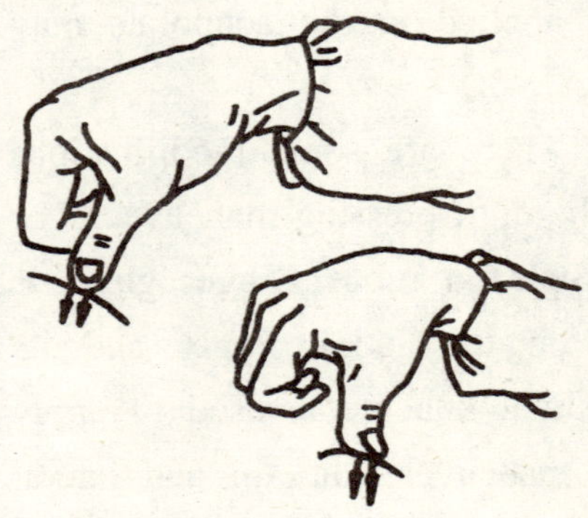

Fig. 3-1 Pressing maneuver

There are some modifications of the pressing maneuver, such as the simultaneous application of pressure by both hands or by one hand with the support of the other hand. No matter how this maneuver is modified, the requirements of therapy are more important than the elegance of movement.

Indications: The pressing maneuver is usually applied to the acupoints or areas on a flat part of the hand or foot to deliver deep pressure without hindering or interfering with the nearby or underlying bones. It can be used with a kneading maneuver in combination. This maneuver can be used to treat continuous dull pain anyplace on the body and chronic diseases, and to maintain health.

2. Digit-pressing maneuver:

Manipulation: The tip or knuckle of thumb and the proximal knuckle of index finger may be used to apply a pressure to the acupoints or areas in a more limited space and with a heavier force to produce a stronger stimulation than in the pressing maneuver. The acupoints for applying pressure must be accurately located without any shift from the correct location through the manipulation, and the strength applied to the acupoints may fluctuate over a wide range (Fig. 3-2)

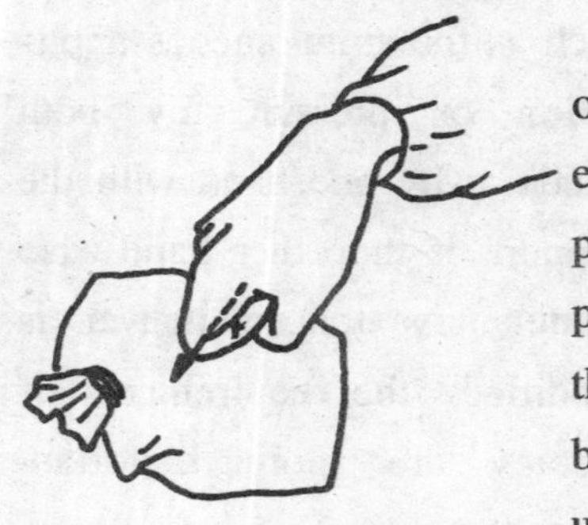

There are some modifications of the digit-pressing maneuver. For example, a rubber finger glove is put on the index finger and its proximal knuckle is used to apply this maneuver; the tip and lateral border of little finger may also be used to apply pressure while it is supported by the thumb and ring finger.

Fig. 3-2 Digit-pressing maneuver

Indications: Digit-pressing is usually applied more forcibly to the fissures of the bones or to more limited spots. It is often used to treat acute or painful diseases.

3. Kneading maneuver:

Manipulation: This maneuver can be divided into finger-kneading and palm-kneading methods. In the finger-kneading maneuver, the pad of the finger is put steadily on the acupoints or areas with the wrist relaxed, and then the forearm is repeatedly swayed to and fro, with the elbow as a fulcrum, to gently and slowly sway and rotate the wrist and palm to conduct the rotating force to the finger. In the palm-kneading maneuver, the thenar and hypothenar prominences or the root of the palm are put over the acupoints or areas for a similar swaying and rotating movement by the forearm. This maneuver should be performed gently and rhythmically (Fig. 3-3).

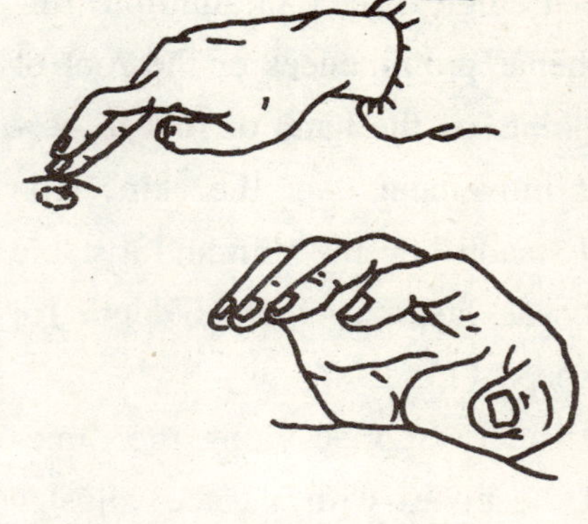

Fig. 3-3 Kneading maneuver

There are some modified methods for doing the kneading maneuver such as using several fingers placed side by side, or with the two palms placed face to face. However, the finger(s) or palm(s) must be placed steadily on the acupoints or areas to gently and persistently apply this maneuver for a longer period of time.

Indications: The kneading maneuver should be applied to the acupoints or areas superficially distributed on a flat and wide region to produce an adjusting and tonic effect. It may be used to treat chronic and deficient diseases, tissue strain, and local swelling and pain. It is also useful for maintaining health.

4. Pushing maneuver:

Manipulation: The pad of a single finger or multiple fingers, and the thenar and hypothenar prominences or the root of palm may be placed at certain points on the hand or foot to perform one directional and linear movement over the skin. The finger or palm should be placed steadily on the skin and a stable pressure applied to reach the tissue layer at a fixed depth for pushing with a slow and even speed (Fig. 3-4).

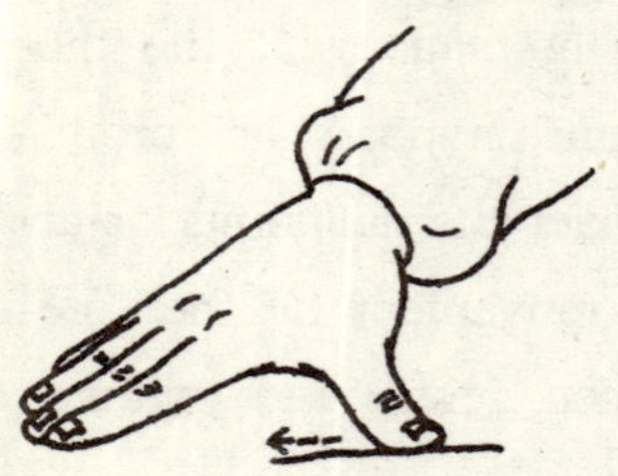

Fig. 3-4 Pushing maneuver

The pushing maneuver is usually applied along the direction of the bones with a force adjusted according to therapeutic requirements. If the pushing maneuver is applied across the bones, the force should be applied to a depth not beyond the most superficial bone, and this force should not be very strong, otherwise the finger or palm will meet resistance, the therapeutic effect may be reduced, and the skin and underlying tissue may be injured.

Indications: The pushing maneuver is usually applied along the longitudinal direction of the fingers and palm or along various sides of the fingers. It is used to treat chronic diseases, suffering due to strain, continuous dull pain and deficient and cold diseases. It is also useful for maintaining health. After application of the pushing maneuver for a period of time, it may be replaced by the rubbing maneuver.

5. Pinching maneuver:

Manipulation: The pinching maneuver is a strong simulating method applied with the tip of thumb and the radial border of the thumbnail to the sensitive acupoints or areas; or applied with the thumbnail edge on one side and the nail edges of the fingers on the other side to apply opposite pressure from both sides. The pinching pressure should be gradually increased to reach the deep tissue and produce a strong stimulating sensation, but the skin should be protected from injury caused by the nails. The pinching maneuver should be applied for a short time and

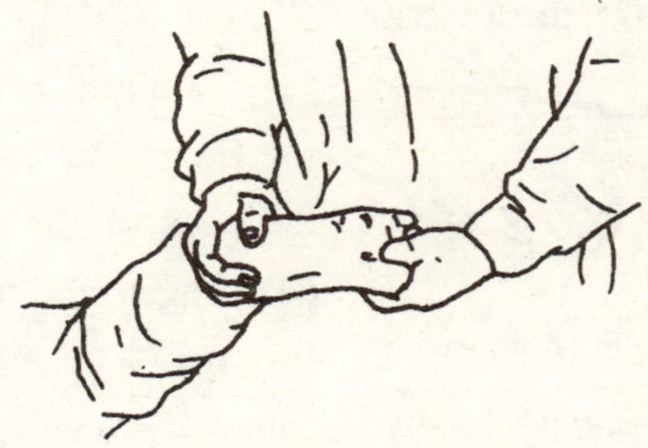

Fig. 3-5 Pinching maneuver at Yongquan (KI 1) acupoint

any discomfort produced by this maneuver can be relieved by the gentle local kneading maneuver. The skin may be damaged if the pinching maneuver is not applied stably with the nails repeatedly slided away from the acupoints (Fig. 3-5).

The tips of both thumbs may be used to employ the opposite pinching maneuver instead of using the nails. The pinching pressure is held for half a minute after it reaches the proper depth, and then the acupoint or area is gently kneaded for half a minute after the pressure is released. The manipulation may be repeated several times, and the pinching maneuver may be applied at a quicker rhythm.

Indications: The pinching maneuver is usually applied at the fingers and toes, at the narrow joint spaces of the fingers and toes, and at the metacarphalangeal joints. It may be used in combination with pressing, kneading and twisting maneuvers to treat acute diseases, pain, psychosis, and neurasthenia.

6. Twisting maneuver:

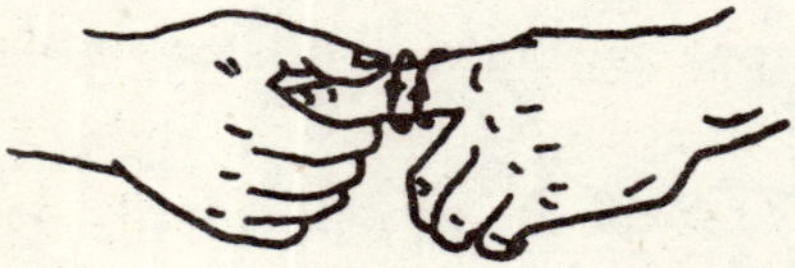

Manipulation: In general, the fingers or toes are held by the pads of the thumb and index finger and twisted to and fro for a certain length of

Fig. 3-6 Twisting maneuver

time. The movement should be quick, smooth, and nimble, without intermission or interruption (Fig. 3-6).

Quick movement is the important requirement for this method, otherwise a slow movement is the kneading maneuver with opposite pads of fingers rather than the twisting maneuver. The manipulation should not be superficial even though it is applied gently; and it should not be sluggish, even if applied forcibly.

Indications: The twisting maneuver is usually applied to fingers, toes, and small joints for treating chronic diseases and local discomfort, and also used to maintain health. It is often in combination with the pinching and pushing maneuvers.

7. Rotating maneuver:

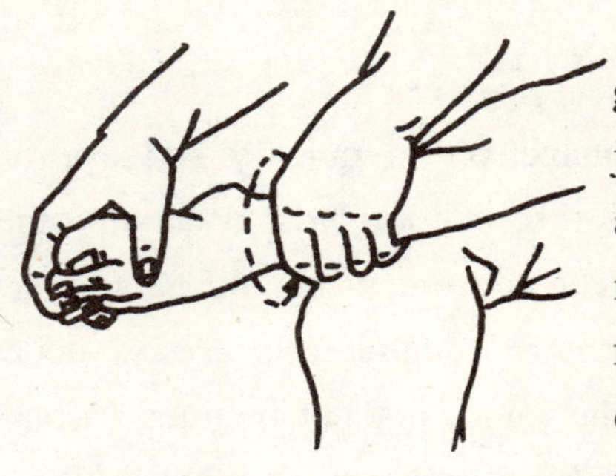

Fig. 3-7 Rotating maneuver

Manipulation: The fingers, toes, wrist, and ankle joints are passively moved in an even, circular rotation. The movement should be gentle, forcible and stable. The range of movement is increased while the speed is decreased until the range of rotation reaches its normal limitation of movement; then the range is gradually decreased and the speed is gradually increased. The movement should be smooth and flexible, and not sluggish or interrupted (Fig. 3-7).

The rotating maneuver can relax and adjust the joints and facilitate their movement. For convenient, safe, flexible and reliable application of this maneuver it can be performed by both hands, one hand for fixation and the other hand for rotation. The rotation should not be applied violently in one direction because this may injure the joint.

Indications: This maneuver is usually applied to the fingers, toes, wrist, and ankle joints to maintain and improve their mobility; and it can also prevent diseases and slow the aging process. It can be used to treat chronic diseases, senile diseases, local injury, and pain. Before applying this maneuver, the joints should be relaxed by pulling and twisting maneuvers to avoid damaging them.

8. Pulling maneuver:

Manipulation: This is a maneuver to quickly and evenly apply traction to one end of the finger, toe, wrist or ankle joint while the other end is fixed. The movement should be nimble and coordinated, but not violent or rough; it is always done along the longitudinal axis of the joint, but not inclined to one side, otherwise the joint and its ligaments may be injured (Fig. 3-8).

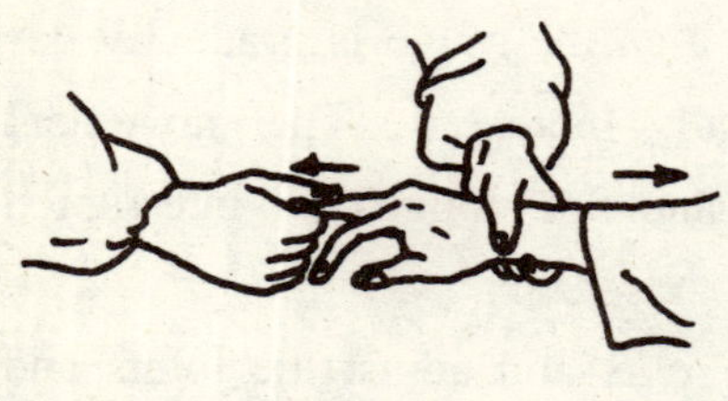

Fig. 3-8 Pulling maneuver

This is a good method to relax the joint, but the click produced in the joint by pulling should not be intentionally induced, because doing this repeatedly may certainly injure the joint.

Indications: This maneuver is applied to the wrist, ankle, interphalangeal, metacarpophalangeal or metatarsophalangeal joints to relax the joints and improve their movement; it can also improve health and slow the aging process. This method can be used to treat senile diseases, local diseases of the joint, and maintain health. It also can be used in combination with the twisting and kneading maneuvers.

9. Rubbing maneuver:

Manipulation: The finger, thenar and/or hypothenar prominence or root of the palm is firmly put at a certain part of the hand or foot to do quick linear movement. To apply the rubbing maneuver, the wrist joint should be naturally extended, the forearm in a horizontal position, the finger, thenar and/or hypothenar prominence or root of palm pressed downward over the skin, and the upper arm repeatedly moved backward and forward with the shoulder joint as its axis. For the finger-rubbing maneuver, the wrist or metacarpophalangeal joint may be used as the axis instead. The to and fro linear movement should be quickly and continuously performed without interruption to produce a hot sensation (Fig. 3-9).

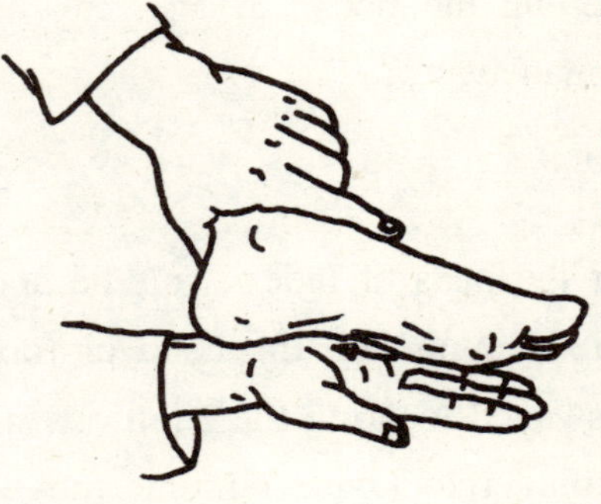

Fig. 3-9 Rubbing maneuver

The rubbing maneuver with a gentle, but not very superficial pressure and a quick rhythm can produce a good effect to promote circulation of qi and blood, relieve stagnation in meridians, expel cold pathogen, and warm and tone the body. The constant rubbing maneuver applied to the sole may particularly produce a marked effect to tone essence and bone marrow, prevent and cure diseases, slow the aging process, and prolong lifes.

Indication: The rubbing maneuver is better to be applied along the bones of the hand and foot, especially on the palm of the hand and sole of the foot to treat chronic diseases, deficient and cold diseases, and mental diseases; and it is also useful for maintaining health and strengthening the body. It also can be used in combination with other maneuvers.

10. Grinding maneuver:

Manipulation: The palm or the pads of index, middle and ring fingers is placed at a certain acupoint on the hand or foot and the wrist joint and arm are swayed to bring the palm or finger pads into a clockwise or counterclockwise circular movement, just like grinding a Chinese ink bar. The cycles of the grinding movement may be gradually increased in diameter centrifugally from the center to the peripheral area, and then gradually reduced in diameter centripetally to the center to produce a hot sensation over this area. The movement should be gentle, the velocity even and coordinated, and the rhythm quick. The pressure of the grinding movement may be gradually and slightly increased, but the quick rhythm should be maintained (Fig. 3-10).

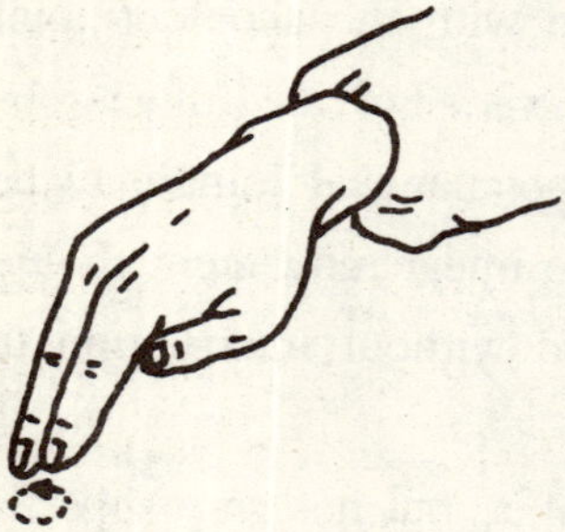

Fig. 3-10 Grinding maneuver

The grinding maneuver is similar to the rubbing maneuver, warming the meridians and removing their stagnation to promote circulation of qi and blood. The grinding movement should be done quickly at an even speed, and the pressure should be maintained to reach a fixed depth. Uneven and sluggish manipulation will not produce the proper effect.

Indications: The grinding maneuver is best performed over a large flat area to treat senile diseases, chronic diseases, and deficient and cold diseases; it is also used to relax local tissue after the heavy grinding maneuver has been applied.

11. Stepping maneuver:

Manipulation: The soles of the patient are stepped upon by the heels or metatarsal and phalangeal part of the physician's foot with rhythmic vibrations. The vibrating movement should be rhythmic and the pressure should be adequately applied depending on the condition of the patient and the nature of disease. However, the physician should not apply his entire cian should not apply his entire

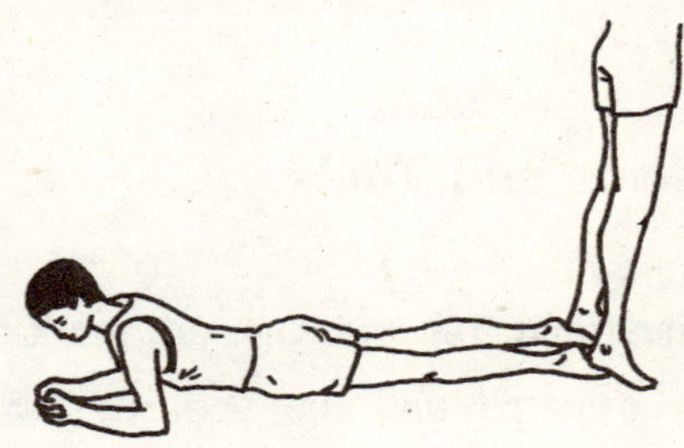

Fig. 3-11 Stepping maneuver

weight on the patient. This is a simple and convenient method for applying pressure over a large area and the physician can save their energy. Constant application of this maneuver is very useful for adjusting the functions of the body (Fig. 3-11).

The stepping maneuver can produce stimulation over a larger area on the anterior and middle part of the sole for adjusting bodily functions, relieving fatigue, refreshing mental activity, and opening the orifices of the sense organs. It also can be used to prevent and treat cerebrovascular diseases.

Indications: The stepping maneuver is useful for treating cerebrovascular diseases, neurasthenia, general fatigue, pain, and traumatic injury with pain; and it can also be used for maintaining health and retarding the aging process. This method also can be mutually applied among family members to prevent and treat diseases.

The essential maneuvers for hand and foot massage have been discussed above. Each of them has its specific use, and they can be flexibly selected and used in combination to improve the therapeutic effect.

II. Supplemental Instruments and Tools

The therapeutic results of hand and foot massage are markedly affected by the maneuvers selected and the skill of the practitioner. Sometimes, an incorrect selection of maneuvers or poor skill may produce an adverse effect. In doing self-massage, supplemental instruments and tools are very helpful, if one has the basic knowledge of the proper techniques. These instruments and tools can help to compensate for less than perfect ability. The supplemental instruments can partially replace the function of the hand in directly performing massage; and the supplemental tools can strengthen and maintain the effects of hand and foot massage. It is worth emphasizing that the supplemental instruments and tools are also very useful in applying hand and foot massage to other people.

The supplemental instruments and tools, including the T-bar, hammer, pestle, massage board, balls and bracelets for maintaining health, and pebble or sand container are discussed as follows. The reader can prepare and modify them for use as needed.

1. Massage T-bar:

Shape and properties: The T-bar look like the handle of a stick. The handle of the bar should be easy to hold firmly with a comfortable feeling, neither too slippery nor too rough. The body of the bar is about 5 cm long and gradually narrows to form a blunt tip, which may be covered with a rubber cap to avoid sliding away from the acupoint when pressure is applied by the bar to the acupoint. The T-bar is best made of hard wood or hard plastic (Fig. 3-12).

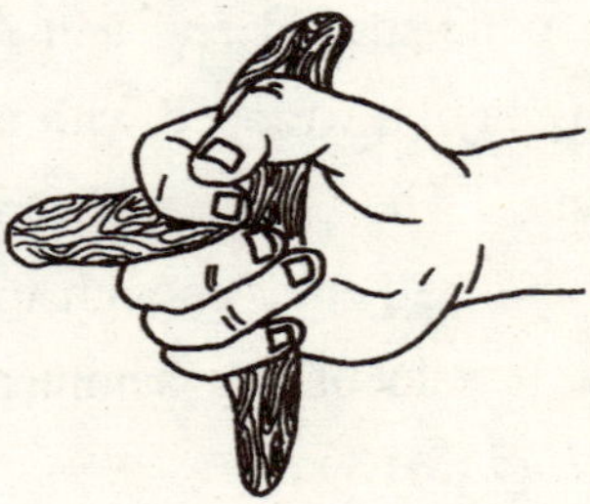

Fig. 3-12 Massage T-bar

Usage: The T-bar can be used as a finger to apply pressing, digit-pressing, finger-pushing and finger-rubbing maneuvers to many places on the hand and foot. The rubbing and pushing maneuvers should be applied along the longitudinal direction of the bones, because rubbing and pushing with the T-bar across the bones may cause local injury if the maneuver is violently applied. The bars may be manufactured in different sizes of various diameters to fit the local anatomical nature of the acupoints or reflecting areas.

2. Massage hammer:

Shape and properties: The massage hammer has a similar

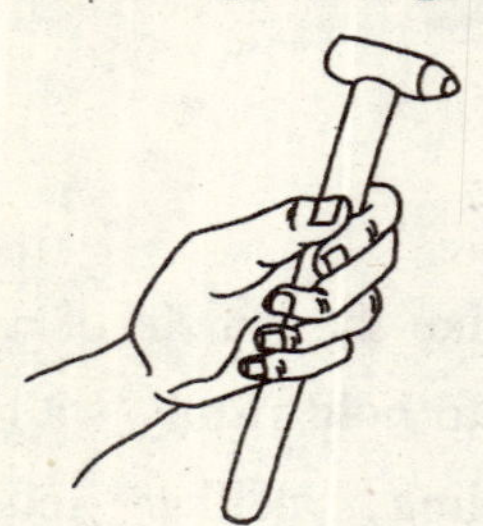

Fig. 3-13 Massage hammer

shape as the common carpenter's hammer. The head of the hammer may be separated from the handle for easy handling by the practitioner. The hammerhead is 1-2 cm in diameter and 4 cm long with a cone-shaped end and a blunt end which may be wrapped with a rubber cushion. The hammerhead should be made of metal or hard wood and be heavy enough to produce the necessary momentum. The handle of the hammer should be slender with good elasticity (Fig. 3-13).

Usage: The massage hammer can take the place of the hand to apply quick knocking, grinding, rubbing, and pushing maneuvers to the acupoints and reflecting areas on the palm of hand and sole of foot. The intensity of force and the frequence of manipulation applied with the hammer should be adequate and even.

3. Massage pestle:

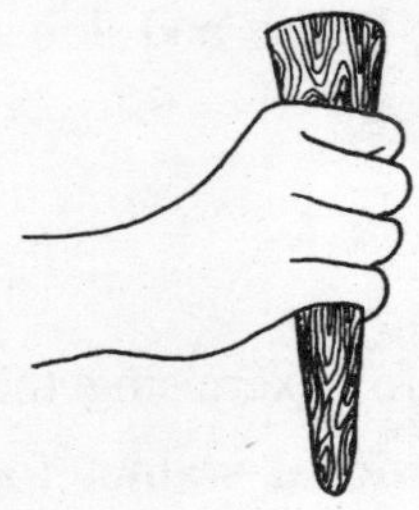

Fig. 3-14 Massage pestle

Shape and properties: The massage pestle is an oval shaped sharpened bar with a wider upper end and a narrower lower end of adequate length for holding in the hand; and 1-2 cm of its upper end may show above the hand. The pestle may be made of smooth stone, wood, or the horn of cattle or sheep (Fig. 3-14).

Usage: After soaking or steaming with a boiled herbal decoction, the hot pestle may be used to push, rub or iron the acupoints over a wide area on the hand and foot. Stone is the best material for the pestle because it can retain more heat energy and better absorb the herbal ingredients. The heat of the pestle should be tolerable for the patient.

4. Massage board:

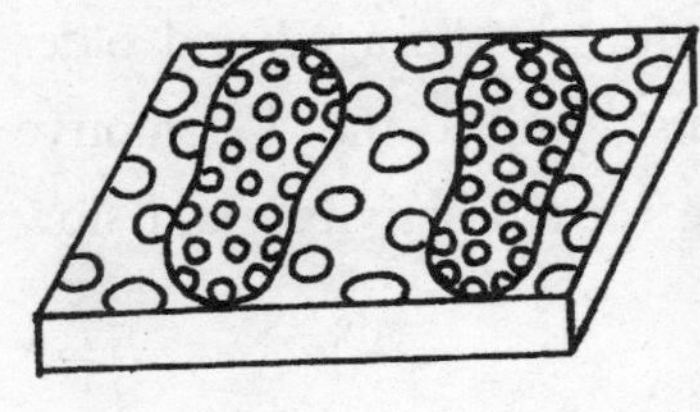

Fig. 3-15 Massage board

Shape and properties: The massage board is made of thick wood or plastic with many protruding papillary eminences carved out from the upper surface of the board in an uneven distribution. The board must be longer than the palm and foot (Fig. 3-15).

Usage: The massage board can be used to perform stepping and kneading or digit-pressing over a wide area of the hand and foot. It is also very useful for maintaining health and doing self-massage.

5. Health balls:

The health ball is a common instrument for exercising the hands, developed and modified from the traditional walnut for

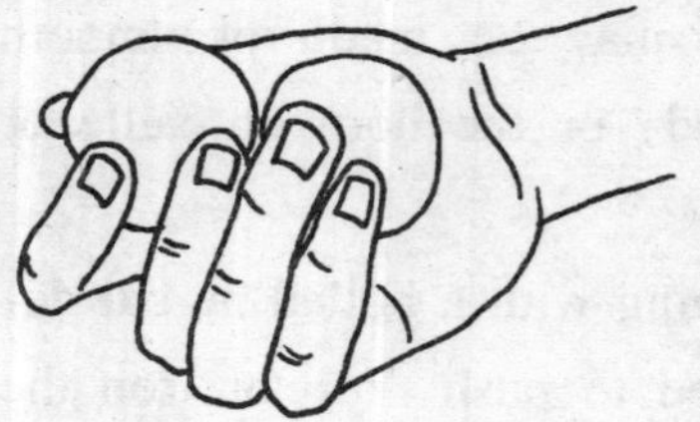

Fig. 3-16 Health balls

hand exercise. The balls are made of crystal, stone, glass, or metal and sold in pairs of different sizes. It is best to choose balls made of natural material for obtaining better results. The balls can be constantly rotated in the palm through the skillful and active movement of the joints to produce a massaging effect (Fig. 3-16). Some people can manipulate as many as 3-5 balls at a time in one hand, or combine the ball exercise with general body exercises.

This is a very helpful exercise for middle-aged and older people to facilitate joint movements, adjust the locomotive function of the whole body, improve mental activity, and slow the aging process.

6. Health bracelet

This is another common instrument for hand exercises. It is a rubber bracelet that comes in different sizes, and is arrayed with small bead-like granules over its outer surface. With the aid of the rebound effect of its elasticity, the user may repeated-

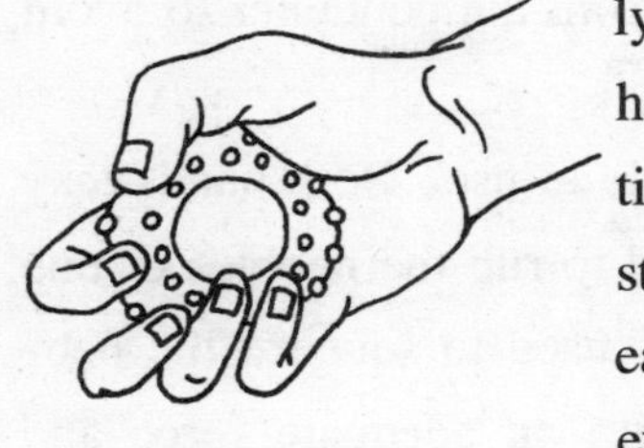

Fig. 3-17

ly squeeze the rubber bracelet as a hand exercise of hand; at the same time, the granules apply pressure to stimulate the acupoints over a wide ar-ea of the palm, producing a massage effect for adjusting and maintaining health (Fig. 3-17). Squeezing the rubber bracelet can also promote the circulation of qi and blood, improve the joint movements, and refresh the mental faculties. Both hands can use the bracelet alternately, and more exercise may be done with the weakest hand. This is a good exercise for youths and people who do mental work and must sit at a desk all day. It is also useful for middle-aged and older people.

When using the exercise bracelet, it is more important to fully squeeze the bracelet each time than to do many repititions. The bracelet can be used anywhere, and persistent exercise can promote growth and development, prevent diseases, retard the aging process, and treat neurasthenia, disturbances of the diges-tive function, and kidney essence deficiency.

7. Pebble container:

This is a wooden box arranged with 3-4 layers of natural round pebbles. It should be big enough to allow an adult to stand on it. A plastic basin may be used instead if a wooden box is not available; and glass balls may be used instead if pebbles from a seashore or riverbank are not available. Broken bits of glass should be carefully removed from the container to avoid damaging the skin (Fig. 3-18).

This instrument is also very simple to use. Both hands may 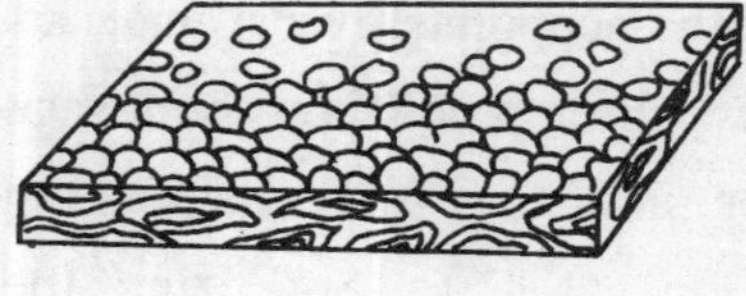 be used to rub the pebbles or one hand is used to squeeze the pebbles with an adequate force and at a proper speed; and the user may stand on the pebbles with bare feet. If this is not tolerable, they may sit on a stool with their feet in the pebbles, and then stand after gradually adapted to it. The process of gradual adaptation is more important for overweight people. If available, it is better to do this exercise in a natural surrounding. The pebbles may be gradually changed from larger to smaller sized, after the user becomes adapted to this exercise.

Fig. 3-18

This is a self-exercise for the hand and foot producing good therapeutic effects. The extent of exercise is adjustable and the pebbles may be boiled or steamed with herbal decoction for even better results.

8. Sand container:

Sand used in building construction or collected from the seashore is put into an adequate container after it is washed clean and sun dried. The sand in the container should be about

5-10 cm deep (Fig. 3-19). Exercise with the sand container is

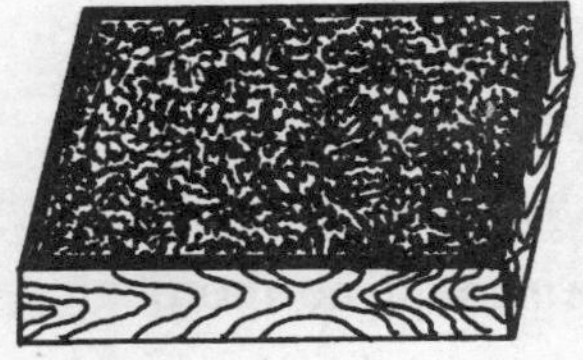

Fig. 3-19 Sand container

similar to that with the pebble container. In addition, the sand may be used to repeatedly rub the foot, especially the spaces between the toes, the joints, and the sole until redness and hotness of the skin is produced. This massage may be carried out at noon or at night to relieve fatigue and produce a sedative and hypnotic effect. It is most useful for chronic patients and senile people with difficulty getting outside. The sand may reused after washing and sun drying.

Besides the supplemental instruments and tools for hand and foot massage mentioned above, there are many ordinary objects around us easily adopted for use if we are familiar with massage principles and techniques. Consistent practice is the important thing for treating chronic diseases and maintenaning health.

III. Massage Preparation and Soaking with Herbal Decoctions

Some preliminary preparation is necessary, and an herbal bath for the hand and foot may be adopted for better therapeutic results, although the effects of the massage alone are reliable.

1. Preliminary preparation before massage:

Preliminary preparation is necessary for both practitioners

and those receiving hand and foot massage.

1) Preparation for practitioners:

(1) The patient's medical history should be carefully reviewed, the present course of the disease should be thoroughly learned, and the patient should be examined in detail to ascertain his general condition and determine if the disease indicates the use of hand and foot massage.

(2) The hands and feet of the patient should be carefully examined to see if they are suitable for massage.

(3) A clean, quiet, warm and comfortable environment must be arranged for massage application and a facility for the easy change of the posture should be provided.

(4) Herbal decoctions and supplemental instruments and tools are prepared if necessary, and the locations of acupoints and reflecting areas must be correctly defined and selected.

(5) The character, method and effects of the massage should be explained to the patient in detail on the first visit in order to earn his trust and cooperation.

(6) For patients with acute and severe diseases, other therapy should be suggested if the hand and foot massage is not effective; and for diseases not indicating this massage, the reasons for selecting other treatment should be patiently explained.

(7) The possibility of difficulties which may occur during treatment should be kept in mind and measures for solving them should be arranged in advance.

2) Patient preparation:

(1) The patient should provide a detailed written or oral health report to the practitioner and cooperate in the physical examination.

(2) For convenience, the patient should thoroughly wash their hands and feet and wear wide and loose-fitting clothes.

(3) An herbal bath should be taken before massage if indicated.

(4) The patient should also listen carefully to the explanation of the massage for sufficient mental preparation.

(5) If the hand and foot massage is not indicated, they should follow the practionioner's advice after gaining an understanding of the situation.

The preparation and requirements for hand and foot massage mentioned above should also be followed for self-massage. The patient may ask a specialist for instruction if they do not know how to prepare, and learn the requirements for hand and foot self-massage.

2. Herbal bath before massage:

This is an important procedure for successful massage, but it is often omitted by many practitioners and patients.

1) Herbal bath proceedure:

(1) Before the herbal bath, the feet, and the legs above the ankle joints, are fully exposed and soaked in water of 50-70

degrees Centigrade, or as high as the patient can tolerate, for 3-5 minutes. The hands are also soaked in hot water, separately. If a facility for hot water soaking of the hands and feet is not available, the hands and feet may be wrapped in hot, wet sterilized towels. Soaking the hands and feet in hot water is itself a good method for maintaining health, besides playing a role as a necessary preparation for herbal bath to allow effective absorbtion of the herbal ingredients.

(2) After soaking the hands and feet in hot water, they are put into a hot herbal decoction for 10 minutes, while the body is relaxed in repose with the eyes closed. The temperature of the decoction may be adjusted according to the patient's tolerance. The softening of the hand and foot skin and the absorption of the herbal ingredients are necessary preparations for an effective massage.

(3) After the herbal bath, the hands and feet are put into clean warm water of 35-55 degrees Centigrade again to wash away the herbal decoction and prepare for the massage.

2) Effects of herbal bath:

The hot-water soak and the herbal bath can have the following benign effects on the body:

(1) The hot water stimulation may promote peripheral blood circulation, adjust metabolism, relieve fatigue, stabilize blood pressure, and improve appearance as well as the quality of sleep and life.

（2）The herbal ingredients are absorbed through the skin, especially through the acupoints and holographic areas on the hand and foot to produce a similar or even better therapeutic effect than oral administration which may cause side effect in the digestive organs. Therefore, it is easily accepted and welcomed by patients.

（3）This method can also improve the adaptation of the hand and foot to changes in the external environment, the respiration of the skin, and the body's comprehensive immunity.

3）Herbal decoction selection:

Following the principles of herb selection for oral administration and the safe and stable absorption of herbal ingredients through the skin, four kinds of herbal decoction are introduced as follows for readers' reference to their selection and use. The recipes were created by the authors through their clinical practice and according to considerations of cost, practicality, convenience, and effectiveness.

（1）Le'an No. 1 recipe:

Composition:

Danggui（Radix Angelicae Sinensis, Chinese angelica）10 gm, Chuanxiong（Rhizoma Ligustici, lovage）10 gm, Honghua（Flos Carthami, safflower）10 gm, Chuanjiao（Pericarpium Zanthoxyli, pepper）10 gm, Huangqi（Radix Astragali seu Hedysari）10 gm, Dahuang（Rhizoma Rhei, rhubarb）10 gm, Chishao（Radix Paeoniae Rubra, red peony）10 gm and fresh ginger 10 gm.

Preparation:

a. The herbs are boiled in 1000 ml of water after soaking for 10 minutes, until 500 ml of decoction is obtained for use.

b. The herbs are wrapped in a cloth bag and soaked in boiled water until the solution cools to an adequate temperature.

Functions and indications:

This recipe can promote blood circulation, relieve stagnation in meridians, tone qi, and stop pain. It can be used to treat diseases of the circulatory, digestive, endocrinal, and reproductive systems. It is especially useful for chronic diseases in adults with general fatigue, cool limbs, stagnation of qi and blood, functional disturbances of the automatic nervous system, cardiac and cerebral-vascular diseases, and chronic diseases of the digestive tract.

(2) Le'an No. 2 recipe:

Composition:

Pugongying (Herba Taraxaci, dandelion) 2 0 gm, Xuchangqing (Radix Cynanchi Paniculati) 10 gm, Machixian (Herba Portulacae, purslane) 10 gm, Longkui (Herba Solani Nigri, nightshade) 10 gm, Rougui (Cortex Cinnamomi, Saigon cinnamon) 15 gm, Dingxiang (Flos Caryophylli, clove) 5 gm, Aiye (Folium Artemisiae Argyi, leaf of mugwort) 10 gm, and Yujin (Radix Curcumae, turmeric) 10 gm.

Preparation:

Same as Le'an No. 1 recipe.

Functions and indications:

This recipe can clear heat and toxic pathogens and adjust qi and consolidate the physique. It also can be used to treat various inflammations, pain, tumors, and cancers due to stagnation of qi and blood, as well as rheumatism, thrombosis, alcoholism, venereal diseases, swelling and pain with unknown causes, and leukemia.

(3) Le'an No. 3 recipe:

Composition:

Kushen (Radix Sophorae Flavescentis, shrubby sophora) 20 gm, Xuanshen (Radix Scrophulariae, figwort) 20 gm, Longdancao (Radix Gentianae, gentian) 10 gm, Dahuang (Rhizoma Rhei, rhubarb) 10 gm, Baizhi (Radix Angelicae Dahuricae, Chinese angelica) 10 gm, Danshen (Radix Salviae Miltiorrhizae, red-rooted sage) 10 gm, Tiannanxing (Rhizoma Arisaematis, jack-in-the-pulpit) 15 gm, and Huanglian (Rhizoma Coptidis, goldthread rhizome) 10 gm.

Preparation:

Same as Le'an No. 1 recipe.

Functions and indications:

This recipe can eliminate dampness, discharge fire pathogens, enrich the blood, and improve facial appearance. It also is used to treat many chronic diseases resistant to other treatments, skin diseases, rheumatic diseases, endocrinal diseases, sequelae of cardiac and cerebral vascular diseases, and extraordinary diseases of unknown origin. It is useful for both expelling pathogens and strengthening and toning the body when used to soak the hands and feet over a long period of time.

(4) Le'an No. 4 recipe:

Composition:

Cebaiye (Cacumen Biotae, arber-vitae) 10 gm, Danzhuye (Herba Lophatheri, lophatherum) 10 gm, Chuanjiao (Pericarpium Zanthoxyli, pepper) 10 gm, Shiye (Folium Kaki, persimmon leaf) 10 gm, Cheqiancao (Herba Plantarinis, common plantain) 10 gm, Guipi (Cortex Cinnamomi, cassia bark) 10 gm, Banxia (Rhizoma Pinelliae, pinellia tuber) 5 gm, and vinegar 5 gm.

Preparation:

Same as Le'an No. 1 recipe.

Functions and indications:

This recipe can enrich Yin, promote the discharge of water, remove impure substance from the body, and promote tissue regeneration. It also can be used to treat diseases in endocrinal, circulatory and locomotive systems, such as diabetes mellitus, obesity, and fatty liver, diseases of the thyroid gland, and hyperosteogeny with deformity. It is especially useful for treating chronic diseases with complications, if applied every day.

A decoction of the above recipes must not be administered by mouth. The dosages of the herbs may vary according to the patient's condition. The patient should consult the practitioner if there is any doubt about using the herbal bath. In addition, the herbal bath should be stopped if skin reactions appear such as an allergic reaction, rhagades, or desquamation. In general, the herbal bath does not cause any harmful side effects if properly administered. The herbal bath is usually applied before hand and foot massage, but the herbs of the above recipes may also be used to prepare cream for massage use. Because of the wide spread use of the herbal foot bath, an electric thermal box was recently invented and produced in China and Japan for the convenient application of the herbal foot bath.

The preparation for massage and the herbal bath needs greater study and investigation for the development of a new therapy.

IV. Precautions and Contraindications

1) Precautions:

(1) The acupoints and reflecting areas and their integrated application, the methods and techniques of manipulation, and the use of supplemental instruments and tools should all be learned well and mastered; and the hand and foot massage should be constantly applied to the patient to obtain the best therapeutic results.

(2) The manipulation pressure should be modified according to the patient, the disease, and the function of acupoints, reflecting areas and maneuvers. This does not mean heavier stimulation necessarily produces a better therapeutic effect or that the heaviest stimulation produces the best result. On the

contrary, an adequate but persistent stimulation may produce a much better therapeutic result. One exception is that in cases of extreme and severe pain stimulation should be increased to the maximum level.

（3）Hand and foot massage is best applied at a fixed time, for example before noon or at night before going to bed. A regular massage should last 20-30 minutes and be done 1-2 times a day. These times may be modified depending on the disease and the condition of the patient.

（4）The hand and foot massage is very useful, but of course not universally effective, and may be used in conjunction with other therapies if necessary.

（5）The safety of this treatment must be ensured and harmful effects corrected before arranging the next session.

2）Contraindications:

（1）The massage is strictly prohibited for hands and feet with marked ulcerations, bleeding, or infectious skin diseases before they are completely cured. It may be applied to the normal hand or foot on one side, even if the other hand or foot is afflicted.

（2）The heavy stimulation is prohibited for acupoints and reflecting areas on the hand and foot of pregnant women, especially for those acupoints and areas related to the female genitalia, but the gentle pressing and kneading maneuvers may be adopted for use.

(3) Hand and foot massage is usually contraindicated for patients with severe heart disease, mental disorders, and hypertension, except for emergency rescue. Even then, only gentle digit-pressing and kneading maneuvers should be applied.

(4) Maneuvers requiring special skill should only be applied by practitioners who have thoroughly mastered them, as any adverse or violent application may damage the hand and foot themselves.

(5) The massage is prohibited for patients with a completely empty stomach, and it is best applied 1-2 hours after eating, except in cases involving abdominal distress caused by food poisoning.

(6) The practitioner's guidance is necessary for the application of hand and foot herbal bath and the decoctions for this therapy must not be administered orally.

The precautions and contraindications mentioned above have been gathered from the clinical experiences of many practitioners over a long period of time for guaranteeing the safety of this therapy. Good therapeutic medical service is assured only after careful analysis and scientific study of diseases and the problems of patients.

CHAPTER 4   DIAGNOSES OF DISEASES AND RESPONSES ON HAND AND FOOT

Besides the function of transmitting stimulation to specific organs and tissues, the acupoints and reflecting areas on the hand and foot can also transmit information about the organs and tissues, especially pathological information for diagnosing and treating diseases. To completely understanding how the hand and foot can be used to make diagnoses, the methods for doing so are discussed as follows:

I. Outline of Diagnosis

Diagnosis is the basis for hand and foot massage. Symptoms can be relieved and diseases can be cured by applying the proper massage to the correspondent acupoints and reflecting areas of the hand and foot only after a correct diagnosis is made by the methods of hand and foot diagnosis. Otherwise, the treatment may be useless, the disease may worsen, and the patient may lose the chance for a cure. This can occur because of oversight in reading positive pathological responses and signs on the hand and foot or by mistaking normal physiological responses for pathological responses.

Four diagnostic methods—inspection, touching, moving, and pressing are discussed as follows:

1. Inspection method:

This is a method of observing the shape, condition, creases and prints, nails, color and luster at different locations on the hand and foot to discover abnormal changes and specific responses for making diagnoses. In general, the diagnostic information can be obtained by observing the general appearance, color, shape, and condition of the hand and foot.

1) Observing general appearances:

In traditional Chinese medicine, this is known as observing "Shen." Shen is the combined appearance of color and luster, but it is difficult to describe in ordinary terms, as it is a mixture of obscure color and blurred luster.

In modern physics, a weak visible light with a wave length of 3800-4200 angstrom (equal to the wave length of blue light) can be irradiated from the body's surface. The brightness of this light is related to the age, sex, physique, and physiological condition of the individual. This is a specific phenomenon showing the body's functional condition. This weak visible light irradiated from the body is similar to Shen described in traditional Chinese medicine, and it may be the scientific explanation for Shen.

In normal people, the hand and foot are bright and moist. The bightness of the skin should be gentle and viable to indicate the richness of essence and blood, and the fullness of spirit and energy described as Deshen (obtaining Shen) in traditional Chinese medicine.

If the hand and foot skin is dull, dry or haggard due to a reduction of luster and moisture, it is called "Shishen" (loss of Shen) in traditional Chinese medicine. This indicates the worsening of diseases, with a poor prognosis and difficult to cure.

If the hand and foot are dark, lusterless, and appear covered with a layer like dark frost, this indicates a reduction of immunity and a high susceptibility to viral influenza, high fever, nephritis, leukemia, tumor or rheumatic fever.

If the dull appearance and reduction of luster occurs in only a localized area of the hand and foot, this indicates the dysfunction of the organ related to this area, producing a serious disease in that organ and a poor prognosis.

The luster of the hand and foot may change with temperature, climate, or emotional and physiological conditions. However, these changes are usually only present in small areas and are of short duration. Therefore, it is important to determine changed general appearances of the hand and foot over a long period of time for correct clinical diagnosis.

In addition, a change in the luster of the hand and foot can also show the development of a disease. As the hand and foot gradually turn brighter and more lusterous and moist, the disease is subsiding to a certain extent and the health of the patient is gradually improved; but as the hand and foot turn gradually darker and less lusterous and dry, the disease is apparently gaining by degrees. This should draw the attention of the practitioner for timely and adequate treatment.

2) Observing color:

This is a method of diagnosis by observing the change of color on different areas of the hand and foot to diagnose diseases in their correspondent related organs.

The observation of color is combined with the observation of Shen (general appearance) in traditional Chinese medicine. Color is an observable change in Shen, and they are mutually correlated. Traditional medical literature says the "increase, decrease, appearance and disappearance of Shen can be shown by the correspondent changes of color." A correct diagnosis can be made only after the observation of both Shen and color in combination.

As with the change of hand and foot luster, color is also constantly being changed by various factors. In clinical practice, the color of the palmar side of the middle pharlanx of the middle finger is considered the "constant color," the standard color for clinical diagnosis.

The colors of the hand and foot can be divided into blue, red, yellow, white, and black.

Blue: Indicates diseases of liver and gallbladder with pain, cold pathogens, stasis of blood, convulsions and chronic injury with pain.

Red: Indicates diseases of heart and small intestine with fever, local inflammation, bleeding, and the early stages of some progressive diseases.

Yellow: Indicates diseases of spleen and stomach with deficient syndrome, damp pathogens, symptoms due to deficiency of trace elements, anemia, and chronic hemorrhage.

White: Indicates diseases of lung and large intestine with deficient syndrome, cold pathogens, pain, and loss of qi and blood.

Black: Indicates deficiency of kidney with cold pathogens, pain, retention of water, blood stasis, and longstanding chronic injuries.

3) Observing shape:

This is a method of diagnosis by observing the changing shape of different parts of the hand and foot. The observation of shape includes the shape of hand, foot, palm, nail, fingers and toes, as well as fingerprints and creases of the fingers, palms and soles. Because of space limitations, it will not be discussed in this chapter.

4) Observing conditions:

If the patients hesitate to show their hands, and their fingers move irregularly and their joints are flexed with a slight tremor, this indicates nervousness. These patients are nervous, sensitive, timid, suspicious, restless and highly irritable people, lacking independence and decisiveness and easily caught in contradictions. Modern medical science has shown that long-standing nervousness may cause functional disturbances of the endocrinal and nervous systems and can produce peptic ulcers, hyperthyroidism, neurasthenia, headache, insomnia, diabetes mellitus, hypertension, coronary heart disease, and even cancer.

Automatic hand tremor indicates lesions in the central nervous system such as parkinsonism and chorea due to rheumatism.

Contraction and stiffness of the fingers indicate hemiplegia of cerebral hemorrhage, thrombosis and embolism, or belong to their prodromal symptoms.

Claw hand or monkey paw is due to injury of ulnar and median nerves, carpal tunnel syndrome, progressive myatrophy, paralysis of median nerve, amyotrophic lateral sclerosis, or poliomyelitis.

Arcuate foot is usually found in nerve paralysis of the lower limbs, bifid spine, or heriditary ataxia.

Flatfoot is usually found in myasthenia, paralysis of the lower limbs, muscular spasms, shortened heel tendon or secondary to knock knee, medial rotation of tibia, and looseness of sole tendons.

The inspecting method should be combined with other methods of diagnosis to avoid misdiagnosis. Abnormal conditions of the hand and foot are usually caused by lesions in the nervous system, but may also be caused by bone fracture, sprain injury, or rheumatoid diseases for differential diagnosis.

2. Touching method:

This is a diagnostic method for examining the temperature, and tactile and pain sensations in the hand and foot.

1) Examination of temperature:

The temperature of the hand and foot is adjusted by both the central nervous system and other specific body structures. Therefore, a change of temperature in the hand or foot is more marked than on other parts of the body.

Hand and foot temperatue may be adjusted by the feedback nerve impulses from the central nervous system and local specific structures when the body is affected by high fever, cold, irritation, depression and fury, or attacked by virus, pathogens or metabolic products. Hand and foot temperature also may be changed when functional body balance is disturbed.

The tip of the index finger is used to detect temperature changes at different parts of the hand and foot because the tip of the index finger is very sensitive to these changes. The normal body temperature is taken as the standard when evaluating temperature changes in the hand and foot. Sometimes this gives only a rough idea about the change of temperature, because it is much less sensitive than a thermometer. However, it is very convenient to use.

The sequence for examining temperature is from distal to proximal end and from radial to ulnar side of fingers; from peripheral to central part of palm and sole; from palm or sole to dorsum of hand or foot; and from left side to right side of hand and foot.

An increase of local temperature on the hand and foot indicates infection, inflammation or progression of a pathological process to its climax in the correspondent organ of that area; and a decrease of local temperature indicates an attack of cold pathogens to the correspondent organ, or the deficiency of Yang in that organ. For example, an attack of cold pathogens in the upper abdominal region may cause coldness and pain as well as chronic diseases in this region, including chronic gastritis, ptosis of the stomach, and chronic nephritis.

If the hand and foot temperature in an individual is always higher than normal this usually indicates the person suffers from hyperthyroidism, hemorrhage in pons, febrile diseases, hypertension, diabetes mellitus, rheumatoid arthritis, or polycythemia.

If the temperature of hand and foot is always lower than normal this usually indicates they are suffering from shock, hypothyroidism, obstruction, stenosis or compression of artery, syringomyelia, scleroderma, dermatomyositis, disseminated lupus erythematosus, Raynaud's disease, cervical rib syndrome, or heart failure.

If the decrease of temperature is limited to the peripheral part of the hand and foot, this indicates the vital energy of the patient is not completely exhausted and the disease is still curable; but if the central part of the palm or sole is very cold, with pale color and cold sweat, this indicates the exhaustion of vital energy with syncope, impotence, and diarrhea.

2) Examination of superficial sensation:

Pain, temperature and tactile sensations should be examined and analyzed in combination for clinical diagnosis. A hot or cold substance, or pin and bone needle are used to touch or scratch the skin to produce sensations and determine the lesion on the correspondent segment of nerve innervation over the affected skin of the hand and foot.

The thumb, thenar prominence, and radial side of the index finger of the hand are innervated by the 6th cervical spinal nerve (C6), the middle finger is innervated by the 7th cervical spinal nerve (C7), the ulnar side of the ring finger, little finger, and hypothenar prominence are innervated by the 8th cervical spinal nerve (C8). A disturbance of cutaneous sensation on the hand indicates a lesion on C6 to C8 spinal nerves. For example, patients with diseases of the cervical spinal column often show a disturbance of sensation on their hands. The discovery of the area with disturbed sensation may show the segment of injured or compressed nerve and provide treatment indications.

The medial portion of the dorsum and sole of foot is innervated by the 4th and 5th lumbar spinal nerves (L4 and L5), and the lateral portion of foot is innervated by the 1st to 3rd lumbar spinal nerves (L1 to L3). The disturbed area of skin on the foot may indicate the location of the lesion in the lumbar and sacral region, such as the prolapse of lumbar intervertebral disc, proliferative osteo-arthritis, and tumor of cauda equina.

As a clue, in patients with a subjective sensation of numbness in the hand and foot, this may be the prodromal symptom of cerebral thrombosis, even though the examination of cutaneous sensation is normal. These patients should have a thorough physical examination to obtain an early diagnosis and determine treatment.

This is a method of diagnosis by examining the active and passive movement of the hand and foot joints, especially the joints of the fingers and toes.

1) Examination of active movement:

When the wrist joint assumes a neutral position, the range of active movement of this joint is flexion to 50-60 degrees, dorsiflexion to 40 degrees, deviation to ulnar side to 30 degrees, and deviation to radial side to 15 degrees (Fig.

4-1).

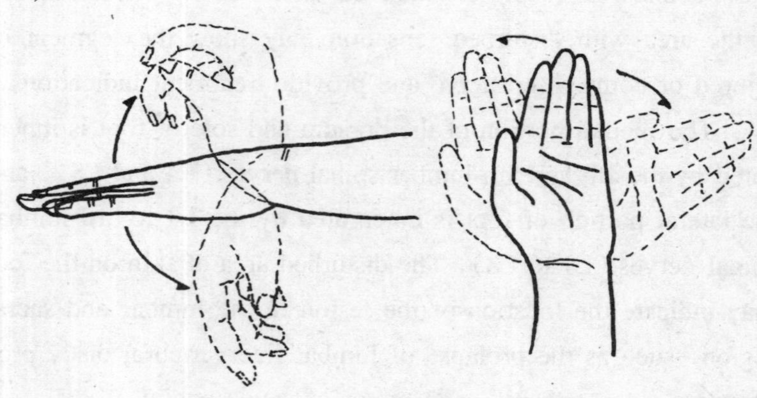

Fig. 4-1 Examination of wrist joint movement

3. Moving method:

When the fingers are extended in a neutral position, the range of active movement of the metacarpophalangeal joints are flexion to 90 degrees and dorsi-flextion to 0 degree or within a small angle, and some degree of medial and lateral deviation. The range of active movement of the proximal interphalangeal joints is flexion to 120 degrees, and the movement of the distal interphalangeal joints is flexion to 60 degrees.

Particular to human beings is the very flexible movement of the carpometacarpal joint of the thumb. When the thumb assumes a neutral position with its ulnar border kept in contact with the radial border of the index finger, it may dorsi-flex as the palm is pressed flat on a table; it can also flex to assume an opposing posture with the palm; and it can again adduct and abduct (Fig. 4-2).

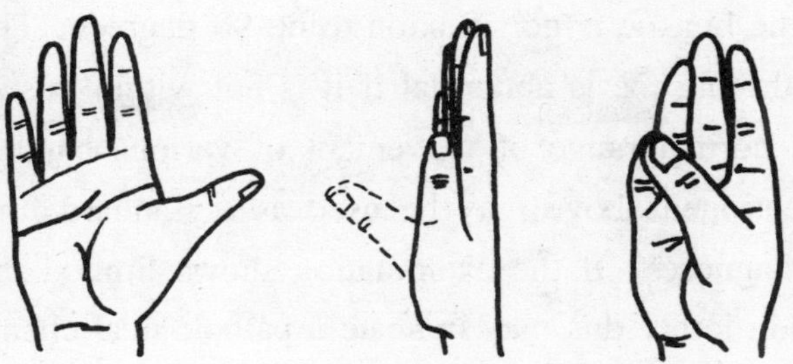

Fig. 4-2 Examination of thumb movement

When the foot assumes a neutral position with the sole perpendicular to the longitudinal axis of the leg, the ankle joint can dorsi-flex to 40-50 degrees, plantarly flex to 20-30 degrees, invert to 35 degrees, and evert to 35 degrees as a combined movement with the subtalar joint (Fig. 4-3).

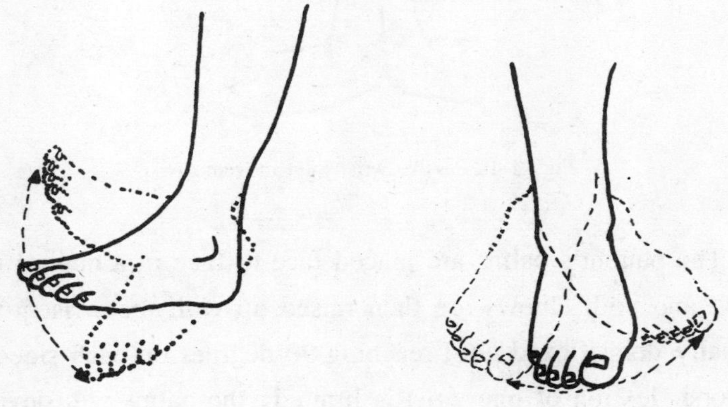

Fig. 4-3 Examination of ankle joint movement

The normal range of movement of the metatarsophalangeal joint of the big toe is dorsiflexion to 60-90 degrees. The movement of the big toe is abnormal if it is not within this range.

The normal range of movement of various hand and foot joints mentioned above may be used as a standard for making clinical diagnoses. If the examination shows limited movement of a certain joint, this may indicate a pathological change in the local structure or its correspondent organ, and a diagnosis can be made in combination with other diagnostic methods.

2) Examination of passive movement:

(1) Comparative examination of passive wrist movement:

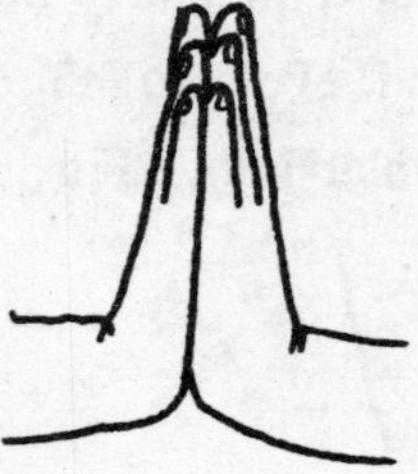

Fig. 4-4a Passive wrist joint movement

The patient's palms are placed face to face in a neutral position, and both elbows are then raised up with the wrist joints gradually dorsi-flexed until reaching 90 degrees on each side. If the dorsi-flextion of one wrist is limited, the palms will deviate to the normal side at an angle greater than 90 degree between the forearm and palm of the abnormal side (Fig. 4-4a).

For examination of palmar flexion of the wrist joint, the dorsum of the hands are put face to face in a neutral position, and are then gradually raised until both forearms are on a horizontal level and an angle of 90 degree is formed between palm 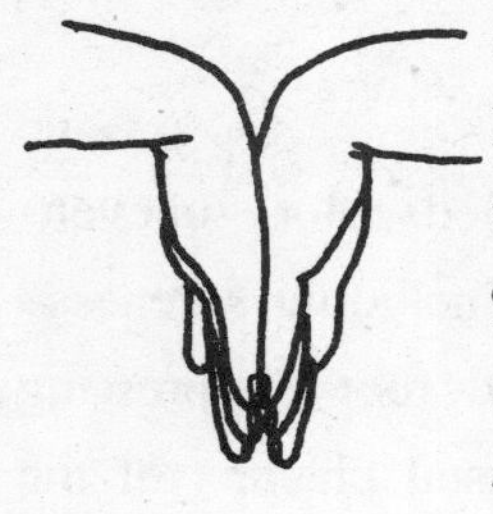 and forearm. If palmar flexion of the hand is limited on one side, the hands will deviate to the normal side, at an angle greater than 90 degree on the abnormal side between the dorsum of the hand and the forearm (Fig. 4-4b).

Fig. 4-4b   Limitation of palmar flexion of the hand with pricking or explosive pain indicates carpal tunnel syndrome or a fracture of the lunar bone.

(2) Examination of passive movement of ankle joint：

The heel of the patient is held in one hand of the practitioner and the instep is held in the other to plantarly flex, dorsiflex, invert and evert the foot. The range of movement of each foot is examined for limitation of movement.

If the range of invertion is too large and the ankle joint is very loose, this may be due to malnutrition on laceration of lateral collateral ligament of ankle joint; if the range of movement is reduced by a stiff joint, or the patient refuses this examination, this may be due to local pain caused by hyperosteogeny of the ankle joint or bursitis.

The moving method of examination can be used not only for diagnosing locomotive disturbances of the hand and foot, but also for general diseases of the body. The diagnosis of a disease in the correspondent organs and tissue can be made by combining other diagnostic methods with the observation of flexibility, movability, stiffness, and locked joints.

4. Pressing method:

This is a technique for finding concealed color, unevenness, and nodules and abnormal sensations including soreness, numb distension, and pain in the hand and foot by pressing them with the pad or radial border of the distal phalanx of the thumb. The sequence of examination is from the proximal end to the distal end, along a vertical direction, and then along a horizontal direction, and from hand to foot.

Concealed color can be observed after the local skin and underlying tissue are pressed by finger as the superficial color fades away. If the concealed color is fresh red, this indicates good health with normal functions of the internal organs; if the concealed red color is pale or dull, this indicates the early stage of disease without symptoms, or an inflammation in the correspondent organ. If the concealed color is normal and the original superficial color can be quickly restored after the release of pressure, this indicates that the vital energy is rich and vatality is exuberant; if the original color is only slowly restored, this indicates that the body is weak and qi and blood are insufficient. If the concealed color is abnormal and the original superficial color can be quickly restored, this indicates that the disease is still in the early stage, the body's resistance is not much impaired, and the disease can be easily cured; and if the original color is only slowly restored, this indicates a chronic disease with a long clinical history.

If a depression is found at the spleen and kidney reflecting areas when the pressing method is applied at the holographic points and areas this indicates the possibility of a congenital single kidney or the removal of the spleen or one kidney by surgery, if sandy nodules are found on the gallbladder, kidney or urinary bladder reflecting area, this indicates the presence of stones in those organs. A movable mass with persistent abnormal feeling indicates the possible presence of a tumor in the body, and a diagnosis of tumor can be made after evaluating the age, physique, and sex of the patient.

An abnormal feeling induced by the pressing method also indicates the presence of pathological lesions. A sore and numb feeling indicates chronic and deficient diseases; numbness indicates stubborn diseases or diseases of the nervous or circulatory system; and distention and pain indicates the presence of inflammation or febrile diseases. If an abnormal sensation is simultaneously present on both hands, the chance for an accuracy diagnosis is much higher.

Among these four diagnostic methods, the inspecting method is the principal technique while the hand examination is most convenient. Therefore, they are the principal methods of diagnosis worth mastering and practicing.

II. Correspondent Responses of Diseases on Hand

For convenient learning, the nail and palm diagnosis techniques with the most specific diagnostic value are discussed in the following:

1. Nail diagnosis

Information about the health of the body can be obtained by observing, touching, pressing, and moving the nail, subungual tissue (nail matrix) and the conjunction of nail and skin. The value of nail diagnosis is briefly discussed as follows:

1) Normal nail:

Shape: The normal nail is an elliptic, ball-shaped plate with a small vertical and horizontal curvature. It has the proper thickness, an elastic hardness, a concealed pink color and a smooth, shiny, and semi-transparent appearance. The lunar zone is normal. The nail fold at the junction of the nail root and skin is red, smooth, soft and regular. There are no ridges or fissures on the surface of the nail plate and no stripes or petechiae on the subungual tissue. The soft red color may be quickly restored after pressure is applied and then released from the nail plate (Fig. 4-5).

Indication: These indicate that both qi and blood are sufficient, meridians are clear, the function of the organs is normal, the body is healthy, and vital energy is plentiful.

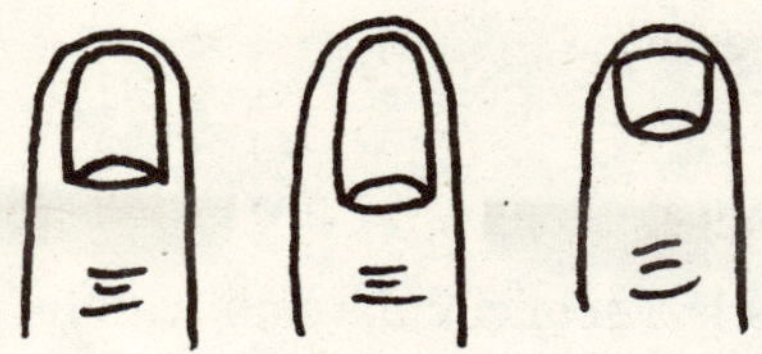

Fig. 4-5 Normal, long, and short nails

2) Long nail:

Shape: The nail plate is bright and clean, but longer than normal and scattered with fine vertical grooves. The subungual tissue is bright, but slightly pale, and the lunar zone is normal. Sometimes, a small hangnail may appear in the nail groove (Fig. 4-5).

Indication: This indicates the impairment of respiratory function, dysfunction of stomach and intestine, and an unsteady emotional condition.

3) Short nail:

Shape: The nail plate is shorter than normal and occupies only one-third of the distal phalanx of finger. The color of the nail plate and subungual tissue is normal and the lunar zone is very small or hiddened underneath the nail fold (Fig. 4-5).

Indication: People with short nails are healthy and robust with a good bursting strength (strength instantly released). Their emotional condition is unstable. People with short nails are easily annoyed, quick to anger, and susceptible to hypertension and liver disease.

4) Round nail:

Shape: This is a semicircular nail with its peripheral borde-

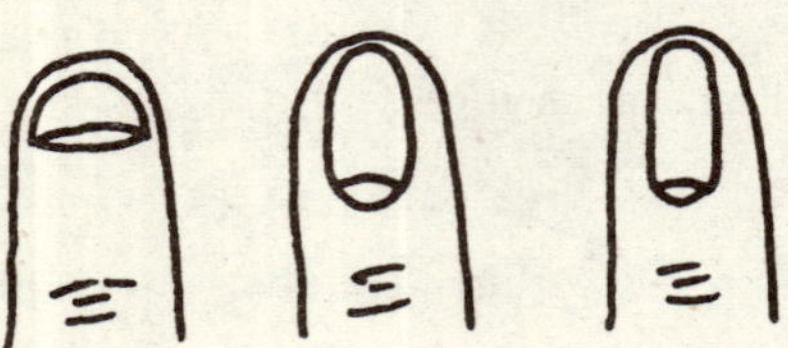
Fig. 4-6 Round, oval and narrow nails

rs coincident with the edge of the distal phalanx, except the proximal border. The nail fold is irregular, but the color of the nail plate and subungual tissue is normal (Fig. 4-6).

Indication: People with round nails have a strong physique, good bursting strength, and an unstable emotional condition, and are susceptible to vertigo, migraine, and metabolic diseases.

5) Oval nail:

Shape: This nail is a small oval plate with normal color and some fine vertical lines visible against the light. The color of subungual tissue is normal and the lunar zone is also normal (Fig. 4-6).

Indication: People with oval nails are healthy, but their emotional makeup is unstable with strong unsatisfied desires. They are susceptible to stomach diseases, headache, and insomnia.

6) Narrow nail:

Shape: The nail plate is narrow and occupys only one-third

the width of the distal phalanx of finger. The skin fold beside the nail is almost as wide as the nail plate. The nail color is uneven and with careful observation some fine horizontal lines are visible on the nail plate. (Fig. 4-6).

Indication: People with narrow nails are susceptible to cervical and lumbar spinal column diseases, hyperosteogeny, and heart disease.

7) Broad nail:

Shape: This nail plate is broad with a much wider free margin. The nail root is depressed and the lunar zone is a narrow stripe. Some vertical and horizontal lines are visible against light. The nail color and subungual tissue are normal (Fig. 4-7).

Indication: People with broad nails are susceptible to thyroid gland dysfunction and sterility.

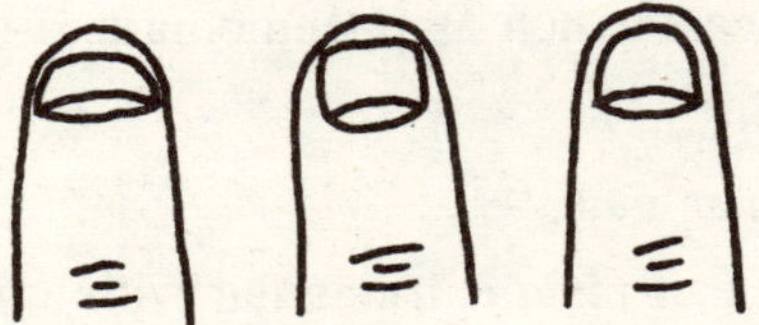

Fig. 4-7 Broad, square, and ladder-shaped nails

8) Square nail:

Shape: The nail plate is square with a transverse diameter narrower than that of the broad nail, and its vertical length is less than one-half of the distal phalanx of finger. The nail plate color, subungual tissue, and lunar zone are all normal. Sometimes red spots may be found on the surface of the nail plate with red and purple colors mutually intermingled in the subungual tissue (Fig. 4-7).

Indication: People with square nails are susceptible to cardiovascular diseases, especially heart diseases.

9) Ladder-shaped nail:

Shape: The free margin of nail plate is narrower than that of the nail root, but the nail's vertical length is normal. Therefore, the nail assumes a ladder shape. The nail plate color, subungual tissue, and lunar zone are all normal. Sometimes the lunar zone also may be in a ladder or triangular shape (Fig. 4-7).

Indication: People with ladder-shaped nails are susceptible to respiratory diseases such as pneumonia and bronchitis.

10) Triangular nail:

Shape: The nail plate is triangular with a wider free margin and a narrower nail root. The nail plate color and subungual tissue are normal. Sometimes the subungual tissue is a white and purple color. The recovery of original color in the subungual tissue is slow after pressure applied to the nail plate is released (Fig. 4-8).

Indication: People with triangular nails are susceptible to

cerebral hemorrhage and thrombosis.

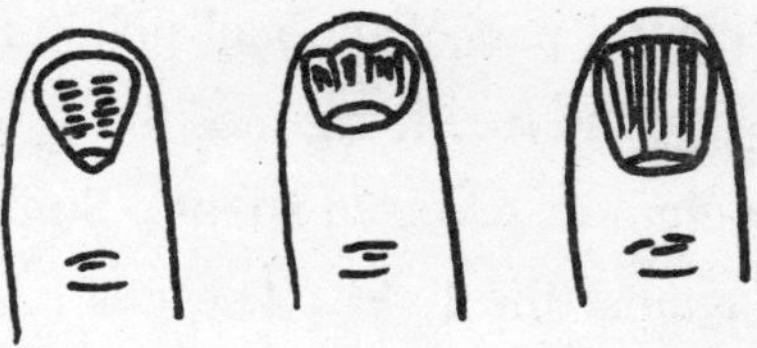

Fig. 4-8 Triangular nail, ingrown nail, and nail with vertical grooves

11) Ingrown nail:

Shape: The bilateral borders of the nail plate, sometimes with a small hangnail, may grow into the nearby soft tissue. The nail is less transparent and the lunar zone is irregular (Fig. 4-8).

Indication: People with ingrown nails are susceptible to dysfunction of the nervous and circulatory systems such as neurasthenia, dysfunction of vegetative nervous system, and congenital heart disease.

12) Nail with vertical grooves:

Shape: The nail plate is uneven and notched with several vertical grooves (Fig. 4-8).

Indication: This indicates deficiency of qi and blood, deficiency of liver and kidney, and an upward attack of liver Yang. These people are susceptible to malnutrition, allergies, and metabolic and respiratory diseases.

13) Convex nail:

Shape: The central part of the nail plate is convex over the peripheral section and the free margin of the nail is curved to the palmar side like a clam or reversed spoon. Some pits on the nail plate are visible against the light. The color of nail plate and subungual tissue is pale, and the lunar zone color is more pink (Fig. 4-9)

Indication: People with convex nails are susceptible to tuberculosis, especially those with a purple nail root.

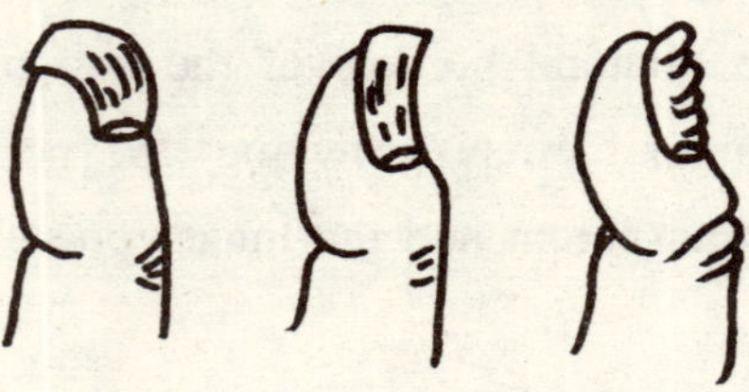

Fig. 4-9 Convex nail, concave nail, and nail with horizontal grooves

14) Concave nail:

Shape: The central part of the nail plate is depressed below the peripheral section and some pits and vertical lines on the nail plate can be observed. The color of the subungual tissue is uneven (Fig. 4-9).

Indication: This indicates liver and kidney dysfunction and susceptibility to infertility with fatigue and low vitality.

15) Nail with horizontal grooves:

Shape: Several horizontal grooves can be seen on the nail

plate, so that it is uneven and its transparence is reduced (Fig. 4-9).

Indication: This indicates liver dysfunction, stagnation of liver qi, susceptibility to hair loss, depression, and dysfunction of the endocrinal system. Petechiae on the subungual tissue are usually caused by trauma.

16) Spoon nail:

Shape: The free margin of the nail is curved to the dorsal side, assuming a spoon shape, and the lateral border of the nail plate splits easily. The color of the subungual tissue is pale, the nail fold is irregular, and some white spots may appear on the nail plate (Fig. 4-10).

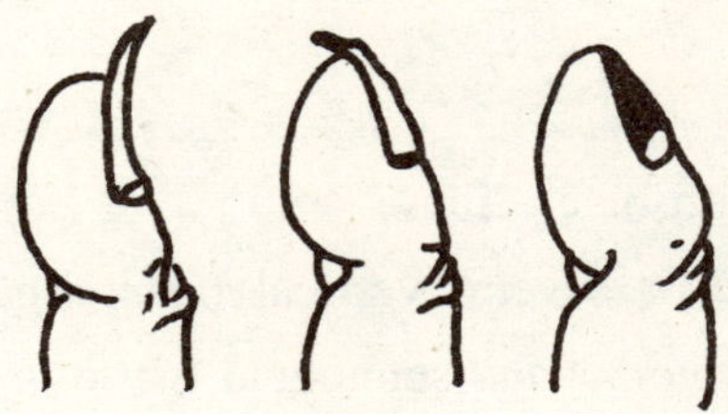

Fig. 4-10 Spoon nail, soft and thin nail, and stripped nail

Indication: This is a manifestation of anemia and malnutrition.

17) Soft and thin nail:

Shape: The nail plate is thin and soft and its resistance and protective function reduced. The color of the subungual tissue is pale and the lunar zone and nail fold are irregular (Fig. 4-10).

Indication: People with soft and thin nails are susceptible to hemorrhagic diseases and calcium deficiency. It is also a manifestation of chronic diseases.

18) Stripped nail:

Shape: The nail plate is stripped from the free margin to the proximal section of the nail bed, like the stripped bark of a bamboo shoot. The nail plate is soft, thin, lusterless and greyish white (Fig. 4-10).

Indication: This indicates susceptibility to hemorrhagic diseases such as digestive tract hemorrhage and anemia due to malnutrition.

19) Nail with black lines:

Shape: One or several vertical black lines appear on the nail plate. The color of the subungual tissue is uneven, the nail fold is irregular, and the lunar zone is dark red and shifted to one side (Fig. 4-11).

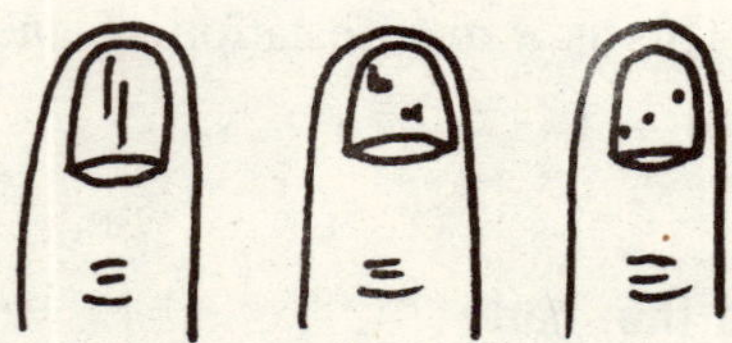

Fig. 4-11 Nails with black lines, and white or red spots

Indication: This indicates dysfunction of the endocrinal system, irregular menstruation, and dysmenorrhea or exhaustion of mental or physical energy.

20) Nail with white spots:

Shape: The small white opaque spots usually appear on all the nails of the hands. On the hands of children they are cloudy white spots (Fig. 4-11).

Indication: This indicates the presence of digestive diseases, and dysfunction of the endocrinal or digestive system. It may appear in children with intestinal parasites. The white pinpoint spots or mixed white and red spots in the central part of the nail indicate ascaris infection.

21) Nail with red spots:

Shape: The red spots appear on the nail plate. A dark purple or whitish red color appears in the subungual tissue. The lunar zone and nail fold are both irregular (Fig. 4-11).

Indication: People with red spots on the nails are susceptible to diseases of the circulatory system such as endocarditis, hemorrhagic diseases, and thrombocytopenia.

22) Spotted nail:

Shape: The nail plate is not smooth and shiny and is scattered with dull yellow spots and unclear vertical lines (Fig. 4-12).

Indication: This indicates the presence of digestive diseases, intestinal parasites, and chronic neurasthenia. People with this condition are easily fatigued.

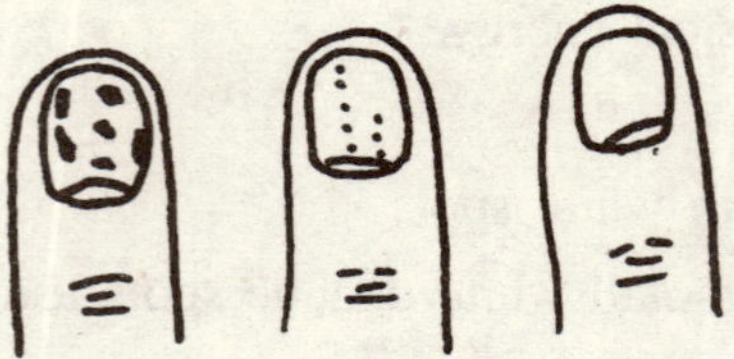

Fig. 4-12 Spotted nail, nail with strings of beads, and nail with
laterally shifted lunar zone

23) Nail with strings of beads:

Shape: The nail plate is covered with strings of protruding beads or scattered with strings of spots in the nail matrix (Fig. 4-12).

Indication: This indicates the presence of malnutrition, impairment of intestinal absorption, deficiency of minute elements, and localized lesions in the digestive tract.

24) Nail with laterally shifted lunar zone:

Shape: The lunar zone is shifted to one side and does not have the shape of a crescent moon. The subungual tissue is an intermingled with dark and pale pink (Fig. 4-12).

Indication: This indicates the exhaustion of physical strength, poor absorption of nutrients, and impairment of body resistance due to exaggerated catabolism.

25) Nail without lunar zone:

Shape: There is no lunar zone on the nail root (Fig. 4-13).

Indication: If the lunar zone is present only on the nail root of thumb and the subungual tissue is pale and dull pink, this indicates that daily life has been disturbed with nervousness, fatique, and impairment of body resistance; and if the lunar zone is absent in all the nails, this indicates susceptibility to circulatory and blood diseases.

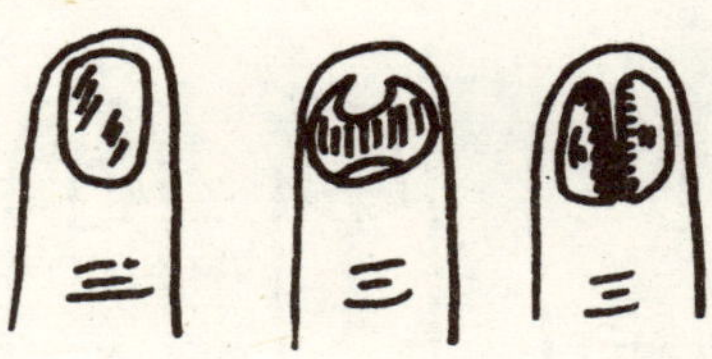

Fig. 4-13 Nail without lunar zone, cylindrical nail, and nail with vertical fissure

26) Cylindrical nail:

Shape: The lateral borders of the nail plate are ingrown forming a cylinder. This is also called tubular nail, like the tubular leaf of a green onion. The pale color of the subungual tissue appearing after pressure is applied to the nail plate may remain for a long time (Fig. 4-13).

Indication: This indicates deficiency of qi and blood and the impairment of body resistance in chronic patients or sedentary people, making them susceptible to serious diseases.

27) Nail with vertical fissure:

Shape: The nail plate is fragile and divided from midline

into two parts (Fig. 4-13).

Indication: This indicates susceptibility to circulatory diseases and dementia. It can also be found in those with trauma, tinea manuum, and chronic diseases.

28) Detached nail:

Shape: The nail plate is detached from the nail bed (Fig. 4-14).

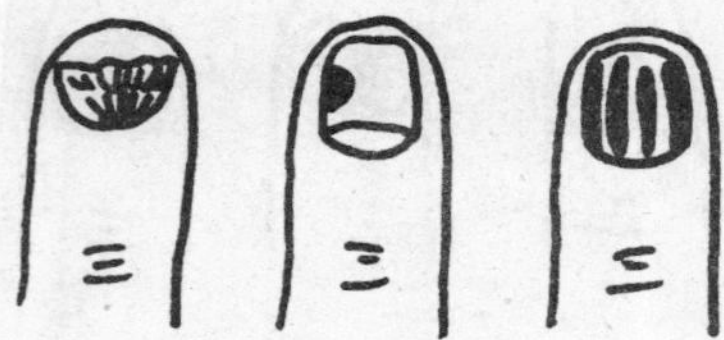

Fig. 4-14 Detached nail, nail with echymosis, and tinea unguium nail

Indication: This is usually caused by pyogenic infection of the fingers. This is also a manifestation of a critical disease called "Jinjue" (destruction of tendons) in traditional Chinese medicine. If the nail does not regenerate, this indicates the patient's extreme weakness caused by the exhaustion of fire in Mingmen.

29) Tinea unguium nail:

Shape: The nail surface is dull, lusterless and rough, and the nail plate is dry, fragile, and yellowish in color like a piece of rotten wood. The nail is thickened on the bilateral borders from the distal end with erosion and defects (Fig. 4-14).

Indication: This condition is caused by impairment of blood circulation, poor nutrition, and an attack of wind and damp pathogens. Those afflicted are susceptible to angitis and muscular atrophy.

30) Nail with echymosis:

Shape: The echymoses in the subungual tissue does not fade away under pressure applied to the nail plate (Fig. 4-14).

Indication: The dark red echymoses indicate a mild injury in the past 3-5 months with a good prognosis; the bluish purple echymoses indicate a recent severe injury or one in the past 1-2 years with a good prognosis; the black echymoses indicate a severe injury in the past 2-5 years with a poor prognosis; and the yellow echymoses indicate an injury over 5 years ago, or a severe injury within a shorter period with a poor prognosis. The spotted echymoses indicate a blunt injury; the striped echymoses indicate a laceration; and the patched echymoses indicate a crushing injury. The nail can be divided into left, right, distal, proximal and central parts to define the location of injury in the correspondent region of the body. The thumbnail represents the head; the index finger nail represents the upper body above the diaphragm; the middle finger nail represents the upper abdomen above the umbilicus; the ring finger nail represents the lower abdomen above the pubic area; and the little finger nail represents the lower body below the pubic area.

The 30 types of nails mentioned above may be used as a

reference, but this method does not produce a conclusive clinical diagnosis. In most patients, several types of nails may be present at the same time. Therefore, a diagnosis can be made only after a comprehensive analysis of the information obtained from nail diagnosis.

2. Palm diagnosis:

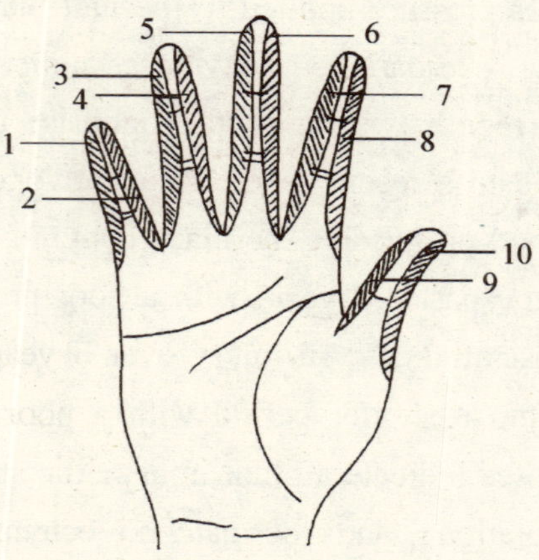

Fig. 4-15a Diagram of palm diagnosis

1-stomach meridian (radial side) 2-spleen meridian (ulnar side) 3-gallbladder meridian (radial side) 4-liver meridian (ulnar side) 5-small intestine meridian (radial side) 6-heart meridian (ulnar side) 7-large intestine meridian (radial side) 8-lung meridian (ulnar side) 9-urinary bladder meridian (radial side) 10-kidney meridian (ulnar side)

This is a method of diagnosis by inspecting, touching, moving, and pressing the comparatively stable diagnostic areas of the palm.

The diagnostic areas on the palm (Fig. 4-15a and 4-15b) have been determined by repeated clinical practice. Most of them are the holographic reflecting areas for treatment, while some others are specific reflecting areas. Four diagnostic techniques are used in combination and the areas with positive responses and the correspondent areas of the diseased internal organs should be carefully examined.

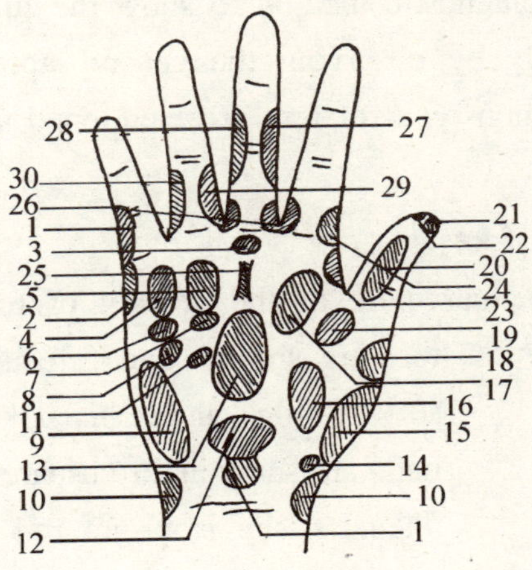

Fig. 4-15b Diagram of palm diagnosis

1-deficiency of qi 2-rectum 3-anus 4-left shoulder 5-dreaminess and fatigue 6-insomnia and fatigue 7-hypertension 8-hypotension 9-constipation 10-cough and asthma 11-reproduction 12-mouth and nose 13-right shoulder 14-right lung 15-left lung 16-esophagus 17-right waist 18-left waist 19-spleen 20-gallbladder 21-abdomen 22-pelvic cavity 23-stomach 24-kidney 25-hemorrhoid 26-rheumatism with edema 27-urinary bladder 28-right heart 29-left heart 30-liver

III. Correspondent Responses of Foot on Diseases

Diagnosis using the foot is similar to that of the hand, although it has some of its own specificity. The general inspection of the foot and big toe are the two important diagnostic methods discussed as follows:

1. General inspection of foot

This is a diagnostic method to show the functional condition of the body by observing the general appearance of the foot. The common types of foot are mentioned as follows:

1) Normal foot:

Shape: The curvature of the dorsum of foot and tips of

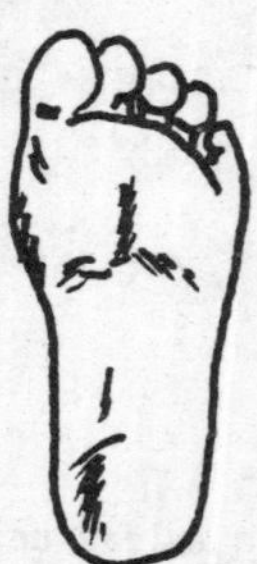

Fig.4-16 Normal foot

toes are smooth and full and the toes are soft, elastic, and regualarly arranged. The nails are shiny and transparent and the subungual tissue is bright red in color. The curve of the arch is normal and smooth. The anterior part of instep, lateral border, and heel pad are regular in shape with no abnormal thickening or atrophy. And there is no tinea infection between the toes (Fig. 4-16).

Indication: This indicates the body is health, built proportionally, and vital energy is rich.

2) Solid foot:

Shape: The foot appears thick and solid, the toes are close to each other, and the big toe deviates laterally. The toenails, arch, and plantar pad are normal (Fig. 4-17).

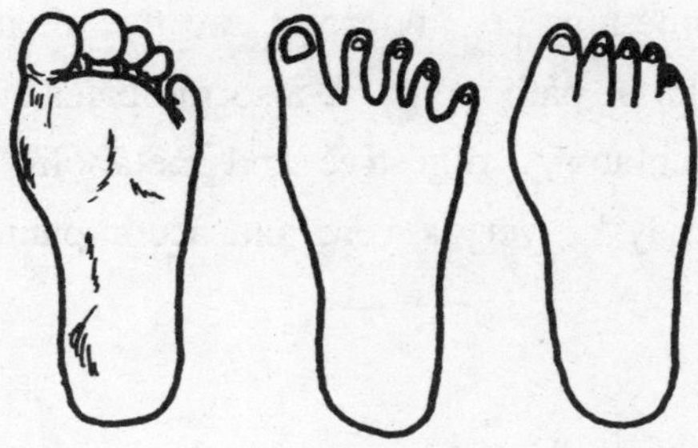

Fig. 4-17 Solid, separated, and drumlike foot

Indication: People with solid feet have normal body functions, are better adapted to the external environment, and can resist attacks of external pathogens. The solid foot has better softness, elasticity and motility, and is usually found in those enjoying good health and long life. If the small joints of the foot are stiff and less mobiles, this indicates susceptibility to vascular diseases of the heart and brain, and spinal nervous system diseases, and if the instep is depressed, it indicates susceptibility to metabolic and liver diseases.

3) Separated foot:

Shape: The foot is thin and the toes are separated from each other. The nails are white with low transparency. The arch is depressed with poor elasticity and the plantar pad is wide (Fig. 4-17).

Indication: This is a type of foot usually found in people with jobs requiring constant standing. It can indicate that the physiological functions are abnormal and the internal organs are subject to attacks of pathogens. It also indicates susceptibility to respiratory, circulatory, digestive and metabolic diseases, and these diseases may be very severe and accompanied by complications.

4) Drumlike foot:

Shape: The big toe is short and narrow and the second toe is protruding. The toes deviate toward the longitudinal midline of the foot to assume a fusiform shape with a wider middle section. The nails are less transparent and the color of subungual tissue is uneven (Fig. 4-17).

Indication: This type of foot is usually caused by wearing ill-fitting shoes causing soreness and pain in the foot, ankle joint, leg, and waist. It also may appear in those with a depressed foot arch, nervousness, schizophrenia, and kidney diseases. These people should pay attention to their emotional state and urinary system.

5) Dry and thin foot:

Shape: The foot is dry, bony and with less flesh. The nails are less shiny and the nail fold is irregular with hangnail

(Fig. 4-18).

Indication: Dry and thin feet usually appear in people with fatigue, especially mental fatigue, exhaustion of vital energy, emotional disturbance, and neurasthenia. They may suffer from headache, general fatigue, sleepiness and poor physical functioning. This type of foot is common in patients with chronic and stubborn diseases.

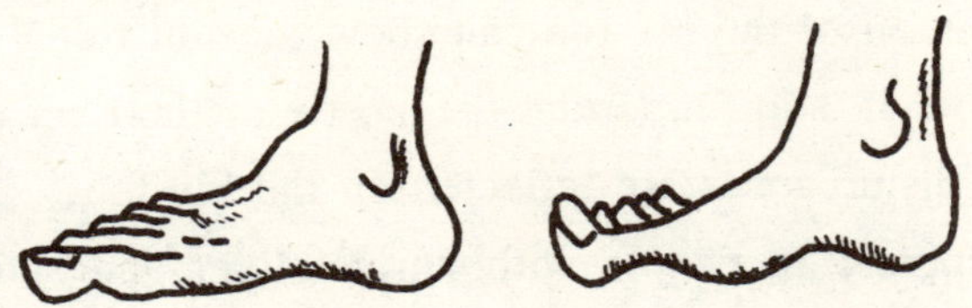

Fig. 4-18 Dry and thin foot and foot with tilted big toe

6) Foot with tilted big toe:

Shape: The big toe is tilted dorsally with the other toes flexed plantarly. The toes are close together, and the veins on dorsum of foot are engorged. The color of subungual tissue of the nails is pale pink or an intermingled pink and white. The first metatarsophalangeal joint is more prominent and the plantar pad is thickened (Fig. 4-18).

Indication: This usually appears in people with mental fatigue or exhaustion of vital energy caused by too much sexual activity. The patient may suffer from dizziness, soreness of waist, tired eyes, impaired blood supply to the eyes, poor adjustment of ciliary muscles, and functional disturbance of the stomach and intestines.

In addition, there are also other types of foot for diagnosis of diseases, and the different types may appear simultaneously in one person. Hand diagnosis and foot diagnosis can be used in combination for the diagnosis of diseases.

2. Inspection of big toe

Inspection of the big toe can show the functional condition of the body. It is an important diagnostic method because many functional disturbances are reflected on the big toe.

In general, in people with normal liver and spleen functions, and who enjoy good health, normal body resistance and rich vital energy, have big toes that are full, plump and red in color. The nail of the big toe is transparent and of a proper thickness, the nail fold and lunar zone are regular, the subungual tissue is normal in color with no dark spots or petechiae, and the big toe is not distorted, the veins are not engorged, and the toe creases are regular.

In individuals with hallux varus (abnormal deviation of big toe to lateral side), if the transparency of the thickened nail is reduced, the lunar zone is deviated to one side, and the nail fold is irregular, this indicates the functional imbalance of the body, exhaustion of vital energy and physical strength, disturbance of digestive functions, neurasthenia, insomnia, or emotional distress.

If the big toe is dry and thin with tendons and bone exposed underneath the skin and toe pad atrophy, and if the nail is dark and dull, the lunar zone absent and the toe pad creases distorted, this indicates an apparent weakness and deficiency of the body and the patient may suffer from chronic and stubborn diseases with a poor prognosis.

If the big toe bulges abnormally and is white or yellow in color, the nail is thin and soft or abnormally thick, the distal border of the lunar zone is surrounded by a purplish red line, the plantar pad (the skin underneath metatarsophalangeal joint) is thickened, and the big toe pad shows wear and tear, this indicates an overload of nutrients in the body and an overburdened heart, liver, and spleen. This usually appears in people with hypertension, heart diseases, cerebrovascular diseases, and fatty liver. These people should control their diet and weight and exercise to improve their health.

3. Pressing foot diagnosis:

The pressing foot diagnosis is another commonly used method. Pressure is applied to certain foot regions by the tip or corner of distal phalanx of thumb or by the knuckle of proximal interphalangeal joint of index finger to produce a sore, numb, distending, or painful sensation to determine the presence of a pathological lesion in its correspondent organ and tissue. The pressure should be applied with a proper and even force. A diagnosis can be made after repeated examination of the sensative spots. The location for the pressing diagnosis is often similar to the reactive therapeutic areas and the biological holographic points. This method is the same as the pressing hand diagnosis, and they can be used in combination.

IV. Relation Between Psychological Factors and Therapeutic Effects

Psychological factors can apparently influence the effects of hand and foot diagnosis and treatment. Good cooperation between practitioner and patients, and active psychological and physical preparation before and after treatment are very useful for curing diseases. In addition, mental relaxation and happiness itself are good therapies. On the other hand, mental distress and depression may induce and cause the worsening of diseases. Psychological factors are equally important in this therapy and in other therapies.

First of all, practitioners are required to be qualified in the application of this therapy so they can quickly and correctly apply the correct manipulation. At the same time, they should maintain a quiet and confident mood when applying treatment, otherwise the patient may lose confidence and patience and the therapy will not produce the desired results. If the practitioner's explanations are ambiguous and not understandable or the manipulation is carelessly and clumsily applied, this will also hamper successful treatment. The patient should continue this therapy over a long time to obtain the best results, because continually changing therapies may produce results contrary to their wishes. At the same time, he may be able to do some self-treatment under proper guidance from the practitioner.

Besides treating the body, the practitioner should also treat the mind, because psychological factors are important in the incidence and development of diseases. Patients may need more mental care than healthy individuals. Under proper instruction, the patient may learn how to adjust his mood, relax the mind, and take life easy for better health. The patient should also try to control bad temper and correct bad habits that are harmful to health and to the course of treatment.

Correct mental care can be a very helpful factor in preventing and treating diseases.

CHAPTER 5 TREATMENT OF COMMON DISEASE BY HAND AND FOOT MASSAGE

In this chapter, treatment for 79 common diseases by hand and foot massage is discussed. Several remarks should be made in advance. First of all, in discussing each disease, general explanations of the illness, acupoints, reflecting areas, and massage methods are all given in some detail. A brief explanation of the disease can help the reader to a general understanding of the disease; the diagrams showing the acupoints and reflecting areas used in treatment may give the reader a rough idea as to the location of these spots, but for their exact location, refer to the detailed description in Chapter 2. Second, in the diagrams of acupoints and reflecting areas, the " • " mark represents digit-pressing maneuver; the "○" mark indicates pressing maneuver; the "ዒ" mark represents kneading maneuver; the "⇑" mark indicates pushing maneuver; the "ⅉ" mark shows rubbing maneuver; the "ᕘ" mark represents grinding maneuver; the "ᖬ" mark shows twisting maneuver; the "ᔦ" mark indicates pinching maneuver; the mark "ᕤ" represents rotating maneuver; the "⊣" mark indicates pulling maneuver; and the "ᖰ"

mark shows stepping maneuver. The "ꙮ" mark represent a combined maneuver of digit-pressing and kneading. Third, some acupoints and reflecting areas listed under each disease may be chozen for one treatment according to the time and place of treatment, and it is not necessary to use all of them at one time. The selected acupoints and areas may be changed day to day, or once every several days.

1. Influenza

Influenza is a common disease of the winter and spring seasons with symptoms of headache, chills, high fever, muscular soreness and pain, nasal obstruction, sneezing, running nose, sore throat, and dry cough with sticky sputum. Babies, aged people, and those with chronic lung diseases may have pneumonia as a complication.

Acupoints and reflecting areas: As shown in Fig. 5-1a and 5-1b.

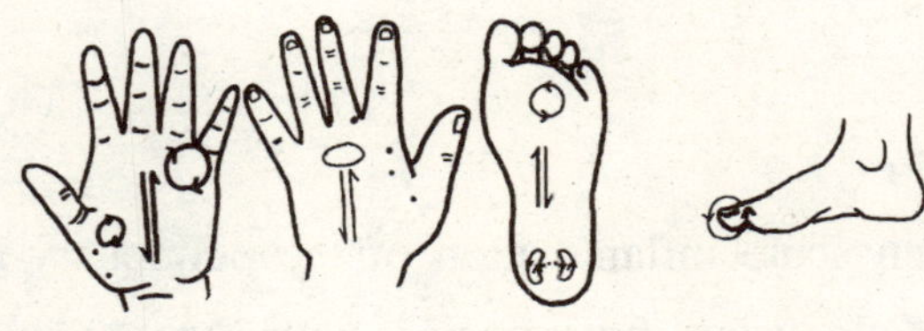

Fig. 5-1a   Fig. 5-1b

Manipulation:

1) Pinching and digit-pressing Yuji (LU 10) and common cold acupoint (EX-PH 25) on palmar side of the hand; Hegu (LI 4), head and lung and heart holographic points on dorsal side of the hand; No. 1 acupoint (EX-PF 4) on plantar side of the foot; and Neiting (ST 44), Qingtou 1 (EX-DF 26) and No. 17 (EX-DF 8) acupoints on dorsal side of the foot.

2) Pressing and kneading maneuvers at lung, pharynx and chest holographic areas on the hand; rubbing central reflecting area of palm and dorsal side of 3rd metacarpal bone; and digit-pressing antifebrile acupoint (EX-DH 43) on dorsal side of the hand.

3) Digit-pressing and kneading lung and head holographic areas on plantar side of the foot and rubbing central reflecting area of sole.

4) The Le'an No. 1 recipe or clear water is used for an herbal bath of the foot, or both the hand and foot. Maneuvers are applied to produce a warm sensation which should be maintained after the bath.

2. Pneumonia

Pneumonia is an acute inflammation of the pulmonary alveoli, caused by diplococcus pneumoniae with symptoms of chill, high fever, chest pain, and cough with rusty sputum. It is a disease common in winter and spring and among people of 20-40 years old.

Acupoints and reflecting areas: As shown in Fig. 5-2a and 5-2b.

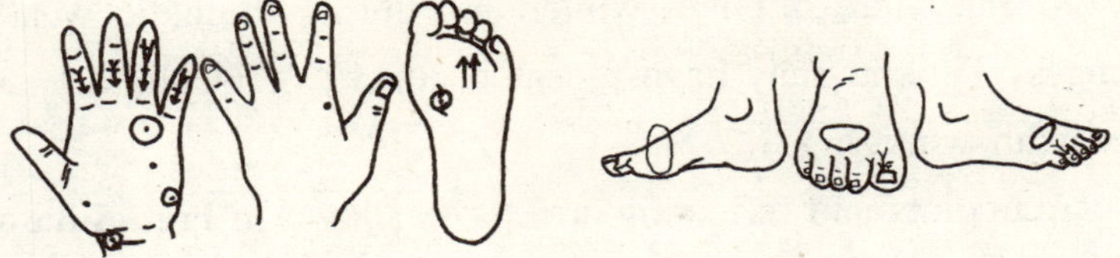

Fig. 5-2a   Fig. 5-2b

Manipulation:

1) Digit-pressing and kneading Taiyuan (LU 9), Yuji (LU 10), Shaofu (HT 8) and lung acupoint (EX-PH 19) on palmar side of the hand; Shaoshang (LU 11) and lung and heart holographic point on dorsal side of the hand; and lung acupoint (EX-PF 28) on plantar side of the foot.

2) Digit-pressing lung reflecting area on the hand and pinching palm, radial and ulnar sides of ring finger and bilateral webs.

3) Pushing reflecting areas of lung and respiratory system on the foot; pinching and digit-pressing dorsal side and tibial and fibular side of big toe, plantar side and tibial and fibular side of 4th toe and bilateral webs.

4) The maneuvers are applied after an herbal foot bath with Le'an No. 2 recipe or clean water. The strong stimulation by hand or supplemental instruments is applied to sensative spots on the foot, and the foot warmth should be maintained.

3. Bronchial Asthma

Bronchial asthma is an allergic disease, appearing in every season, but more often in winter and during dramatic weather changes. Patients may have repeated attacks of inspiratory dyspnea with wheezing.

Acupoints and reflecting areas: As shown in Fig. 5-3a and 5-3b.

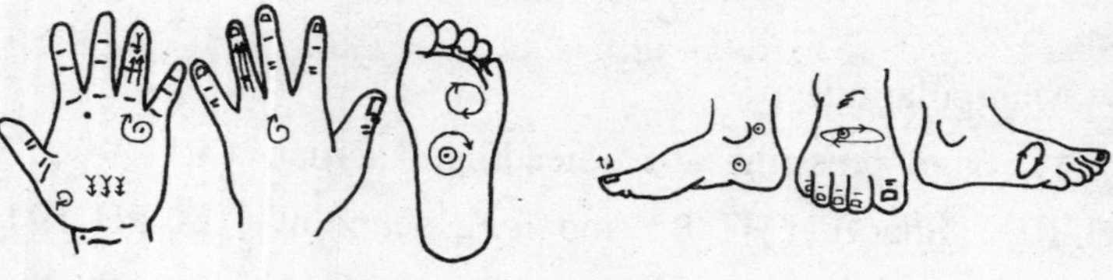

Fig. 5-3a   Fig. 5-3b

Manipulation:

1) Digit-pressing and kneading Taiyuan (LU 9), cough and asthma acupoint (EX-PH 10) and anti-asthmatic acupoint (EX-PH 32) and pinching lung acupoint (EX-PH 19) and 3 Jianli acupoints (EX-PH 31) on palmar side of the hand; and pressing and kneading Shaoshang (LU 11) on dorsal side of the hand.

2) Digit-pressing and kneading No. 7 acupoint (EX-PF 10) on plantar side of the foot; and digit-pressing Taixi (KI 3), No. 17 (EX-DF 18) and No. 29 (EX-DF 20) acupoints on dorsal side of the foot.

3) Grinding lung, pharynx, chest and diaphragm reflecting areas on hand; grinding thenar prominence; and pushing sides of ring finger.

4) Digit-pressing and kneading lung, respiratory system, chest and diaphragm reflecting areas on foot; and twisting and kneading big toe.

5) The maneuvers are applied after the foot bath with clean water; the heavy manipulation is applied at the sensitive spots, and then the medium and gentle manipulation is applied after the symptoms are relieved.

4. Lung Cancer

Primary lung cancer is a malignant tumor of the lung with cough, persistant and severe chest pain, hemoptysis, shortness of breath, fever, and poor appetite.

Acupoints and areas: As shown in Fig. 5-4a and 5-4b.

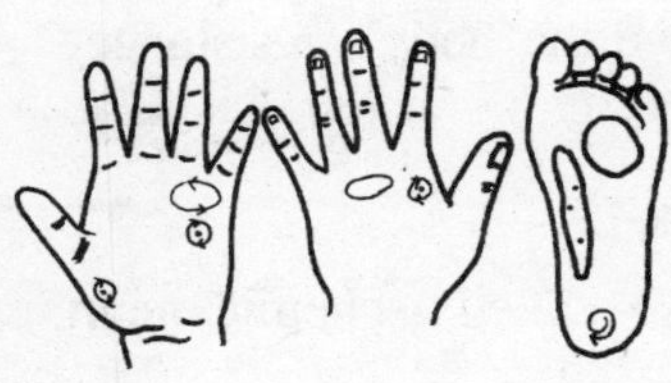

Fig. 5-4a

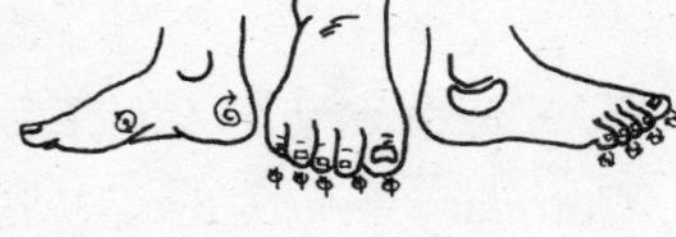

Fig. 5-4b

Manipulation:

1) Heavily digit-pressing and kneading Taiyuan (LU 9),

Yuji (LU 10) and Shaofu (HT 8) on palmar side of the hand and lung and heart holographic point on dorsal side of the hand.

2) Heavily digit-pressing and kneading Jiegen acupoint (EX-DF 23) on medial side of the foot and 3 Aigen acupoints (EX-PF 36 to 38) on plantar side of the foot.

3) Persistently pinching and kneading lung, chest and diaphragm holographic areas on hand; pinching and kneading sides of ring finger and its bilateral webs, more manipulation should be applied to the sensitive spots and positive spots discovered by inspection.

4) Persistently rubbing and digit-pressing lung, lymphatic immunity and cancer zone reflecting areas on foot; twisting and rotating all toes, with extra manipulation of the big toe and 4th toe; and rubbing central region of sole, and grinding heel.

5) The Le'an No. 2 recipe is used to do longer foot baths. A persistent stimulation should be applied to the sensitive areas. The manipulation on spleen and stomach acupoints and reflecting areas may be applied to improve the body's resistance.

5. Coronary Heart Disease

Coronary heart disease is also called ischemic heart disease, and is caused by an imbalance between the coronary blood flow and the blood supply demand of the cardiac muscles, due to the impairment of coronary circulation. Patients may suffer from heart palpitations, cardiac arrhythmia, chest distress, shortness of breath, precordial pain, and nausea and vomiting.

Acupoints and reflecting areas: As shown in Fig. 5-5a and 5-5b.

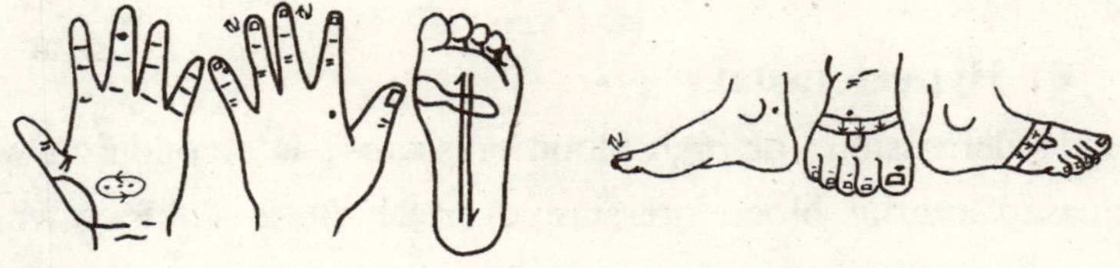

Fig. 5-5a   Fig. 5-5b

Manipulation:

1) Digit-pressing and kneading Shenmen (HT 7), 3 Jianli acupoints (EX-PH 31) and heart acupoint (EX-PH 18) on palmar side of the hand; Shaoshang (LU 11), Shaochong (HT 9), Zhongchong (PC 9) and lung and heart holographic point on dorsal side of the hand.

2) Digit-pressing and kneading Taixi (KI 3) and No. 17 acupoint (EX-DF 8) on dorsal side of the foot.

3) Kneading and pressing heart reflecting area on hand; and twisting and pinching thumb and middle finger.

4) Pushing and pressing heart, chest and diaphragm reflecting areas on the foot; twisting and kneading all toes; and heavily rubbing midline of sole.

5) The Le'an No. 1 recipe is used for longer foot baths. The strong stimulation is applied at the acute stage, and the medium stimulation is applied after the symptoms are relieved.

Acupoints and reflecting areas of the chest, lungs and digestive system may be selected according to the condition of the disease.

6. Hypertension

Hypertension, or high blood pressures, is a condition with increased arterial blood pressure over 21.3/12.7 kPa, which may cause vertigo, headache, distension of head, tinnitus, heart palpitations, numbness of fingers, flushed face, irritability, and insomnia.

Acupoints and reflecting areas: As shown in Fig. 5-6a and 5-6b.

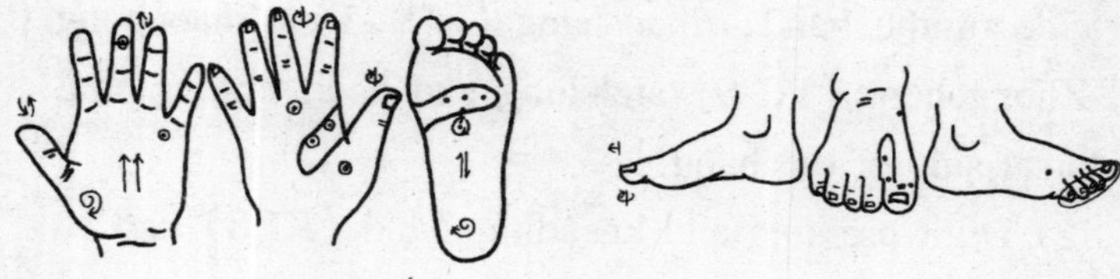

Fig. 5-6a   Fig. 5-6b

Manipulation:

1) Digit-pressing heart (EX-PH 19) and heart palpitation (EX-PH 13) acupoints on palmar side of the hand; Hegu (LI 4), hypotensing (EX-DH 16) and Chaqi (EX-DH 34) acupoints and lung and heart holographic point on dorsal side of the hand.

2) Digit-pressing and kneading Yongquan (KI 1) and heart (EX-PF 29), liver (EX-PF 32), kidney (EX-PF 33) and gall-bladder (EX-PF 34) acupoints on plantar side of the foot; and Xiaxi (GB 43) and hypotensing (EX-DF 4), No. 16 (EX-DF 7), No. 22 (EX-DF 13) and No. 23 (EX-DF 14) acupoints on dorsal side of the foot.

3) Pushing and grinding central part of palm and heart holographic area on the hand; and twisting and rotating all fingers, especially the thumb and middle finger.

4) Pressing and kneading heart and head holographic areas on the foot; rotating and pulling all toes; rubbing central part of sole of the foot; grinding heel of the foot; and pushing dorsal space between 1st and 2nd metatarsal bones.

5) The Le'an No. 1 recipe may be used for foot bath. The acupoints and reflecting areas of kidney and abdomen may be selected according to the disease and the medium stimulation is applied.

7. Hypotension

If the blood pressure is lower than 12/8 kPa, the condition is called hypotension, or low blood pressure, and the patient may suffer from dizziness, tinnitus, vertigo, weakness, shortness of breath, cool hand and foot, spontaneous sweating, sweating at night, and nausea, vomiting, and syncope in severe cases.

Acupoints and reflecting areas: As shown in Fig. 5-7a and 5-7b.

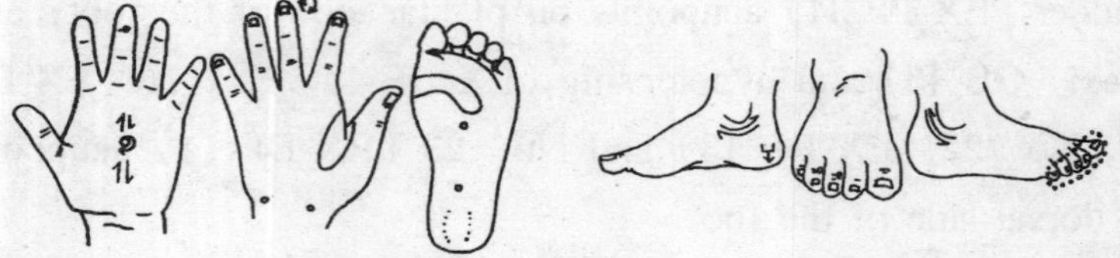

Fig. 5-7a   Fig. 5-7b

Manipulation:

1) Pressing and kneading Yanggu (SI 5) and hypertensing acupoint (EX-DH 13) on dorsal side of the hand; and heart acupoint (EX-PH 18) on palmar side of the hand.

2) Digit-pressing Yongquan (KI 1) and No. 3 acupoint (EX-PF 6) on plantar side of the foot; and No. 26 (EX-DF 17) and Qingtou 2 (EX-DF 27) acupoints on dorsal side of the foot.

3) Quickly rubbing palm, and pinching and twisting sides of middle finger.

4) Digit-pressing and kneading heel, head, and heart holographic areas on foot; rubbing central part of sole, heel, and medial and lateral malleoli until producing a warm sensation; and stepping on the heel.

5) The Le'an No. 1 recipe may be used for hand and foot bath. The acupoints and reflecting areas of kidney and spleen may be selected for patients with cool palm and sole until a warm sensation is produced. The heavy manipulation may be

applied to patients with severe symptoms.

8. Heart Palpitations

Heart palpitations are a subjective symptom with fright, restlessness, and loss of self-control. Patients may also suffer from insomnia, poor memmory, vertigo, dreaminess, and tinnitus.

Acupoints and reflecting areas: As shown in Fig. 5-8a and 5-8b.

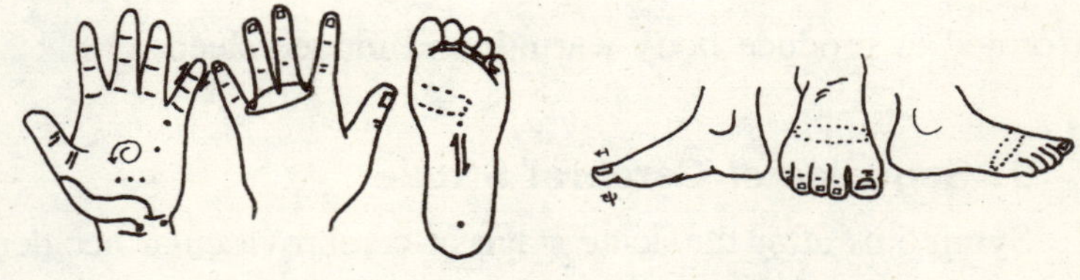

Fig. 5-8aFig. 5-8b

Manipulation:

1) Digit-pressing and kneading Shenmen (HT 7), Shaofu (HT 8), Daling (PC 7) and 3 Jianli acupoints (EX-PH 31) on palmar side of the hand and Shaochong (HT 9) on dorsal side of the hand; and pinching and kneading heart palpitation acupoint (EX-PH 13) on palmar side of the hand.

2) Deeply digit-pressing and kneading Yongquan (KI 1) on plantar side of the foot; and digit-pressing and pinching insomnia acupoint (EX-PF 1) on the heel.

3) Grinding palm; rubbing sides of the little finger until producing a warm sensation; pressing heart and kidney holo-

graphic areas on palmar side of the hand; and digit-pressing central part of the palm.

4) Heavily rubbing the sole; digit-pressing and kneading heart, kidney, chest, and diaphragm holographic areas on plantar side of the foot; pulling and rotating all toes; and pinching pads of toes and metatarsophalangeal joints.

5) The Le'an No. 3 recipe is used for foot bath. Other related acupoints and areas may be selected according to the disease, and the manipulation should be gently and continuously performed to produce body warmth and induce sleep.

9. Sequelae of Cerebral Stroke

Symptoms after the acute stage of cerebrovascular accidents may include hemiplegia, deviation of mouth and eye, disturbance of speech, dripping of saliva from mouth, dysphagia, and numbness of hand and foot.

Acupoints and reflecting areas: As shown in Fig. 5-9a and 5-9b.

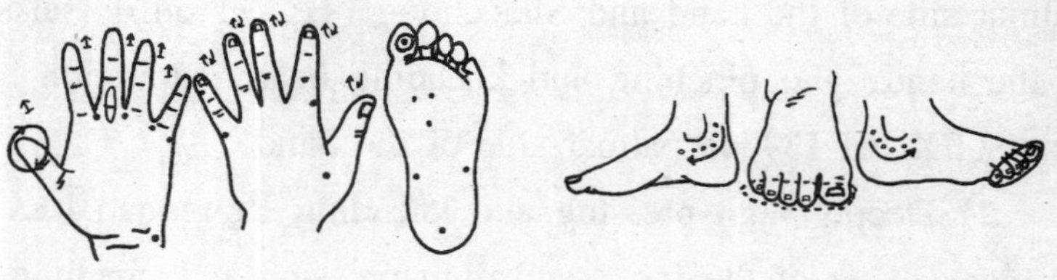

Fig. 5-9a   Fig. 5-9b

Manipulation:

1) Heavily digit-pressing and pinching Shenmen (HT 7)

and 8 palmar acupoints (EX-PH 33) on palmar side of the hand; and Shaoshang (LU 11), Erjian (LI 2), Hegu (LI 4), Shaoze (SI 1) and Qiangu (SI 2) on dorsal side of the hand.

2) Heavily digit-pressing heart (EX-PF 29), liver (EX-PF 32) and kidney (EX-PF 33) acupoints on plantar side of the foot; Shenmai (BL 62) on posterolateral border of the foot; and medial and lateral Ququan (EX-PF 43) on plantar side of the foot and Sibai acupoint (EX-PF 42) at the heel.

3) Continuously digit-pressing and kneading head holographic area on the hand; pinching and kneading radial and ulnar borders and pads of fingers; and twisting and pulling all joints. Greater manipulation is applied to the affected side.

4) Persistently digit-pressing and kneading head holographic area on the foot, pads of toes and central part of the sole; and pushing and pressing medial and lateral malleoli. Greater manipulation is applied to the affected side.

5) The Le'an No. 1 recipe may be used for hand and foot bath before maneuvers are applied. In addition, the pinching and digit-pressing maneuvers can be applied to nail roots of fingers and toes. Other acupoints and reflecting areas may be selected according to the disease.

10. Leukemia

Leukemia is a cancer of the bone marrow characterized by an abnormal increase of white blood cells. Its main symptoms include anemia, fever, hemorrhage, edema, numbness and weakness of limbs, and enlargement of liver, spleen and lymph nodes.

Acupoints and reflecting areas: As shown in Fig. 5-10a and 5-10b.

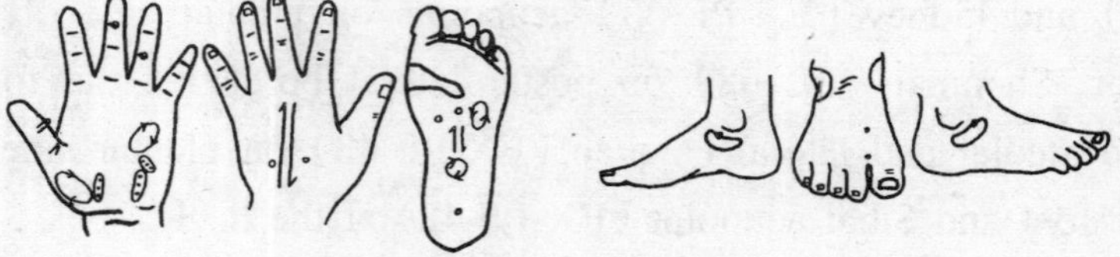

Fig. 5-10a   Fig. 5-10b

Manipulation:

1) Persistently pressing and kneading Daling (PC 7), Laogong (PC 8), Shenmen (HT 7), heart (EX-PH 18), liver (EX-PH 21) and spleen (EX-PH 17) acupoints on palmar side of the hand; and waist and leg pain acupoint (EX-DH 3) on dorsal side of the hand.

2) Continuously pressing and kneading Yongquan (KI 1), Aigen 1 (EX-PF 36), Yongquan (KI 1), and insomnia (EX-PF 1) on plantar side of the foot; and Shangqiu (SP 5), Qiuxu (GB 40), Taichong (LR 3), and Xingjian (LR 2) on dorsal side of the foot.

3) Persistently pressing and kneading heart, liver, spleen and kidney holographic areas on the hand; heavily rubbing central part of palm; and pushing dorsum of the hand.

4) Heavily rubbing central part of sole; digit-pressing and kneading heart, liver, spleen, kidney and lymphatic holograph-

188

ic areas on the foot.

5) The Le'an No. 1 recipe may be used for hand and foot bath. The medium stimulation is applied and greater manipulation may be applied to the sensitive areas. The force of manipulation should not be very violent, or it may cause damage to the skin or a subcutaneous hemorrhage.

11. Anemia

Anemia is a clinical condition with hemoglobin content in blood lower than 120 gm/L in adult men, 110 gm/L in adult women and 100 gm/L in pregnant women. Patients may suffer from pale complexion, shortness of breath, rapid heart beat, diarrhea, amenorrhea, and reduction of sexual desire.

Acupoints and reflecting areas: As shown in Fig. 5-11a and 5-11b.

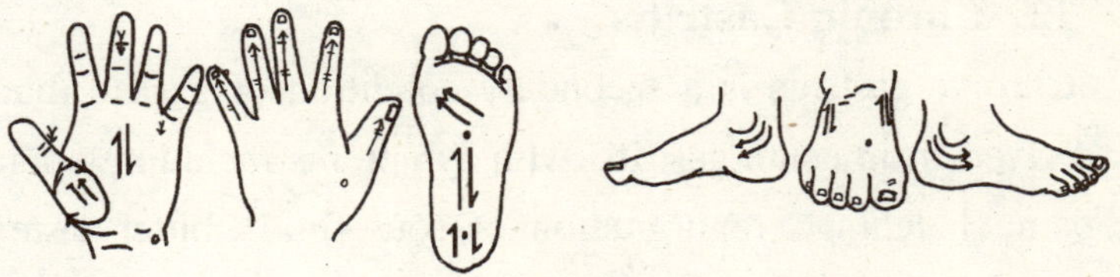

Fig. 5-11a   Fig. 5-11b

Manipulaiton:

1) Continuously pressing and kneading Shenmen (HT 7) on palmar side of the hand and Hegu (LI 4) and Shaochong (HT 9) on dorsal side of the hand; and pinching heart (EX-PH 18), spleen (EX-PH 17) and heart palpitation (EX-PH 13)

acupoints on palmar side of the hand.

2) Persistently digit-pressing and kneading Yongquan (KI 1) and insomnia (EX-PF 1) acupoints on plantar side of the foot; and Taichong (LR 3) on dorsal side of the foot.

3) Pushing and kneading heart holographic area on the hand and sides of all fingers; and rubbing palm.

4) Pushing and pressing heart, spleen, kidney, stomach and intestine holographic areas on the foot; heavily rubbing central part of sole, heel, heel tendon and the conjunctive part of medial and lateral malleoli.

5) The Le'an No. 1 recipe may be used for hand and foot bath. The manipulation should be gently and continuously applied, and other acupoints and reflecting areas may be selected according to the disease.

12. Chronic Gastritis

Chronic gastritis is a secondary condition of gastric mucosa, derived from acute gastritis with symptoms including epigastric pain, belching, regurgitation of sour fluid, bitter taste in mouth, constipation, and fullness in chest and upper abdomen.

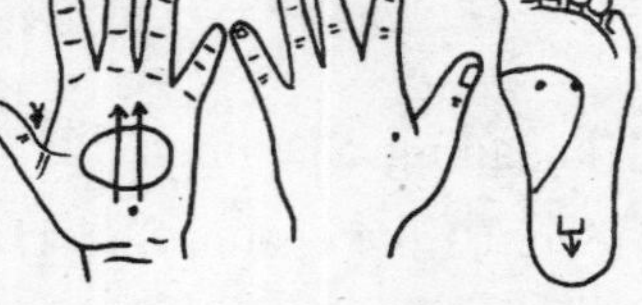

Fig. 5-12a

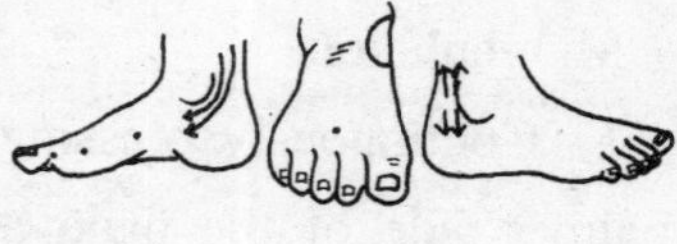

Fig. 5-12b

Acupoints and reflecting areas: As shown in Fig. 5-12a and 5-12b.

Manipulation:

1) Digit-pressing Daling (PC 7), and stomach and intestine pain (EX-PH 8) acupoints on palmar side of the hand and stomach holographic point on dorsal side of the hand; or digit-pressing and pinching spleen acupoint (EX-PH 17) on palmar side of the hand.

2) Digit-pressing pain-controlling (EX-PF 30) and No. 10 (EX-PF 13) on plantar side of the foot; Neiting (ST 44), Dadu (SP 2), Taibai (SP 3) and Gongsun (SP 4) acupoints on dorsal side of the foot; and stomach holographic point on the foot.

3) Pushing and pressing midline of palm; pressing stomach, spleen, and digestive system holographic areas on the hand; and grinding central part of palm.

4) Pressing and grinding stomach, intestine and related lymphatic holographic areas and other reflecting areas of digestive organs on the foot; heavily rubbing central part of sole; and stepping on sole.

5) The Le'an No. 3 recipe can be used for foot bath. It is best to apply medium manipulation. The anus, chest and diaphragm holographic areas can be selected for treatment of constipation and fullness of chest and upper abdomen.

13. Peptic Ulcer of Stomach and Duodenum

The chief symptom of this disease is epigastric pain with

regular and long-lasting periodic attacks. The patient may also suffer from belching, regurgitation of sour fluid, nausea, distending pain in bilateral costal region, and loss of appetite.

Acupoints and reflecting areas: As shown in Fig. 5-13a and 5-13b.

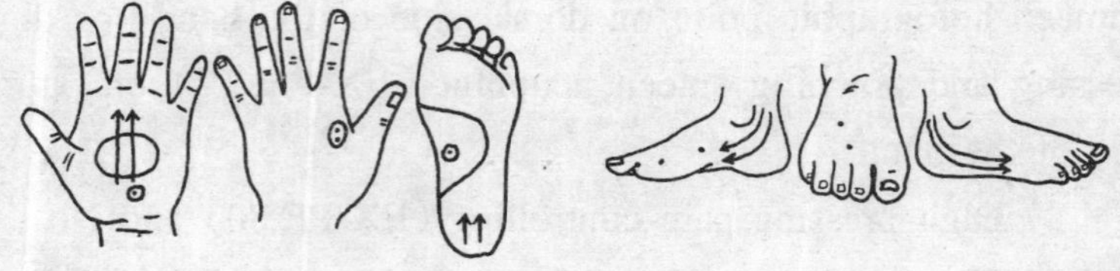

Fig. 5-13a   Fig. 5-13b

Manipulation:

1) Digit-pressing stomach and intestine pain acupoint (EX-PH 8) on palmar side of the hand; and stomach and duodenum holographic points on dorsal side of the hand.

2) Digit-pressing and kneading No. 6 acupoint (EX-PF 9) on plantar side of the foot and No. 19 (EX-DF 10) on dorsal side of the foot, or pinching and kneading Neiting (ST 44), Taibai (SP 3), Gongsun (SP 4) and Dadu (SP 2) acupoints on the foot.

3) Grinding and pushing midline and central part of palm; and pressing stomach, intestine and kidney reflecting areas on the hand.

4) Heavily rubbing sole and medial and lateral borders of the foot; and pressing and kneading holographic areas of stomach, duodenum and other digestive organs on the foot.

5) The Le'an No. 3 recipe can be used for foot bath. The medium stimulation is continuously applied to the sensitive spots and the patient should be placed on a special diet by the practitioner.

14. Gastrointestinal Neurosis

The impairment of digestive function is due to functional disturbance in the higher centers of the nervous system, and the patient may suffer from poor appetite, regurgitation of sour fluid, belching, heartburn, vomiting, increased bowel gurgitation, and abdominal pain, as well as neurasthenia, dreaminess, fatigue, and weakness.

Acupoints and reflecting areas: As shown in Fig. 5-14a and 5-14b.

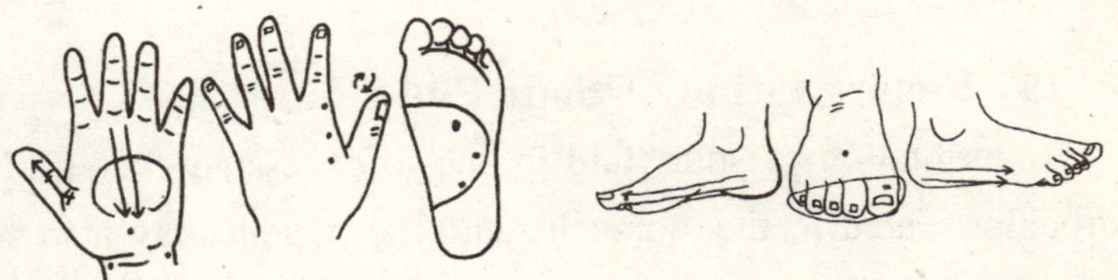

Fig. 5-14a   Fig. 5-14b

Manipulation:

1) Digit-pressing and kneading stomach and intestine pain acupoint (EX-PH 8) on palmar side of the hand, and stomach and head holographic points on dorsal side of the hand; or pinching and pressing Shenmen (HT 7) and Taiyuan (LU 9) on palmar side of the hand and Erjian (LI 2) and Sanjian (LI 3) acupoints on dorsal side of the hand.

2) Digit-pressing and kneading Yongquan (KI 1), No. 8
(EX-PF 11) and No. 3 (EX-PF 6) acupoints on plantar side of
the foot; and Xiangu (ST 43) on dorsal side of the foot.

3) Pressing and kneading stomach and digestive tract holographic areas and pushing heavily and repeatedly from proximal
end of middle finger to wrist joint; or twisting and pinching all
sides of thumb.

4) Pressing and kneading stomach, digestive tract, head,
and spleen reflecting areas on the foot; and the pushing maneuver is applied from heel along medial and lateral borders of the
foot to tips of the big toe and little toe.

5) The Le'an No. 3 recipe can be used for foot bath. The
manipulation should be applied with medium stimulation.

15. Regurgitation of Sour Fluid

Regurgitation of sour fluid is due to excessive excretion of
hydrochloric acid in the stomach, and the patient may also suffer from irritability, dry throat, bitter taste in mouth, distension
of chest and upper abdomen, and belching with foul odor.

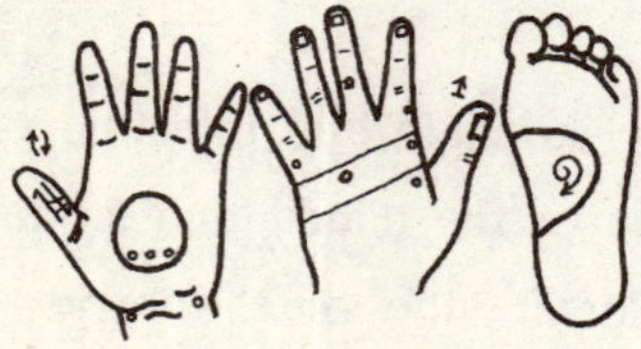

Fig. 5-15a

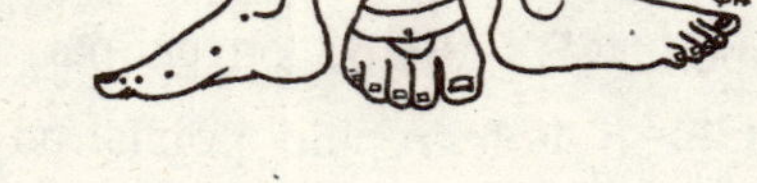

Fig. 5-15b

Acupoints and reflecting areas: As shown in Fig. 5-15a

194

and 5-15b.

Manipulation:

1) Pressing and kneading Shenmen (HT 7), Taiyuan (LU 9), 3 Jianli acupoints (EX-PH 31) and stomach holographic point on palmar side of the hand and Erjian (LI 2), Sanjian (LI 3) or Kongji (LU 6) on dorsal side of the hand; and pinching and digit-pressing Zhongkui (EX-DH 1) on dorsal side of the hand.

2) Digit-pressing and kneading Neiting (ST 44), Yinbai (SP 1), Dadu (SP 2), Taibai (SP 3), Gongsun (SP 4) and Shangqiu (SP 5) acupoints on dorsal side of the foot.

3) Pushing and pressing stomach, digestive tract, chest, and diaphragm holographic areas on the hand; twisting and pulling thumb; and rubbing palm and medial and lateral borders of the hand.

4) Pushing and grinding stomach, digestive tract, chest and diaphragm reflecting areas on the foot; grinding central part of the sole; and pulling and rotating the big toe.

5) The Le'an No. 3 and No. 4 recipes can be used for foot bath. The medium manipulation is applied and other acupoints and reflecting areas may be selected for use.

16. Hiccups

Hiccups are caused by intermittent contraction of the diaphragm due to stimulation of the vagus and phrenic nerves, and the typical symptom is an automatic and quick expiration with a short wheezing noise.

Acupoints and reflecting areas: As shown in Fig. 5-16a and 5-16b.

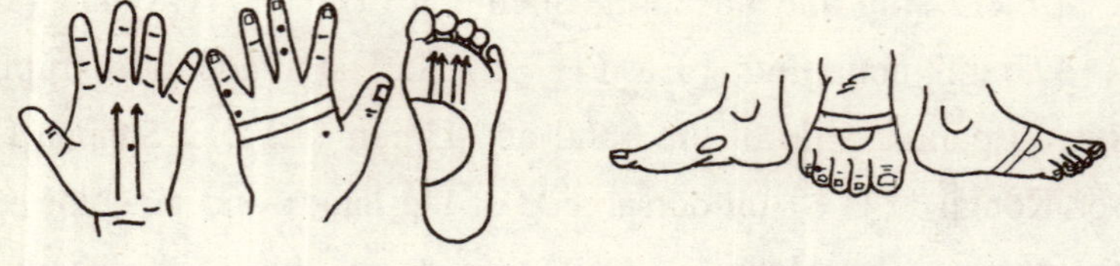

Fig. 5-16a   Fig. 5-16b

Manipulation:

1) Pinching and digit-pressing Laogong (PC 8) on palmar side of the hand and Qiangu (SI 2), Zhongkui (EX-DH 1), occipital headache (EX-DH 6d) and diaphragm (EX-DH 17) acupoints on dorsal side of the hand; and kneading stomach holographic point on the hand.

2) Pinching and digit-pressing Zuqiaoyin acupoint (GB 44) on the foot.

3) Pressing and kneading chest and diaphragm reflecting areas on the hand; and pushing from proximal end of middle finger to palmar carpal crease.

4) Digit-pressing and pressing chest, diaphragm and stomach holographic areas on the foot; pushing deeply the spaces between 1st and 2nd, and between 2nd and 3rd metatarsal bones.

5) The heavy or medium stimulation is applied. Patients with repeated attacks of hiccups over a long time, projectile vomiting, or stiff tongue should be carefully examined to rule out cerebrovascular diseases and brain lesions.

196

17. Neurogenic Vomiting

This is vomiting caused by a stimulation of the central nervous system due to disease or trauma such as cerebral concussion, motion sickness, lesions, hypertension, and Meniere's disease. It may also be caused by drunkenness and anorexia.

Acupoints and reflecting areas: As shown in Fig. 5-17a and 5-17b.

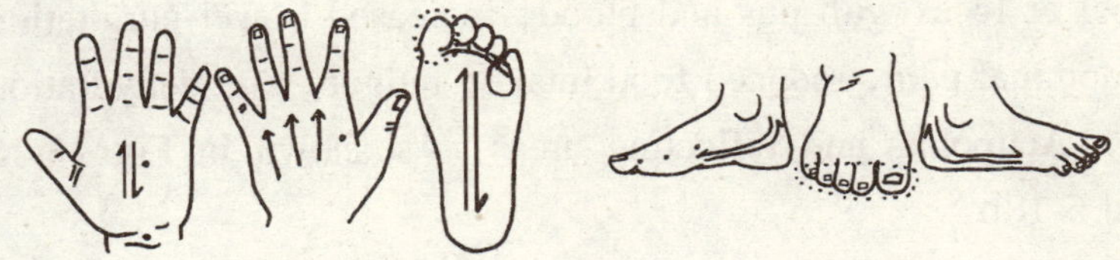

Fig. 5-17a   Fig. 5-17b

Manipulation:

1) Heavily digit-pressing and kneading Laogong (PC 8) on palmar side of the hand and Zhongkui (EX-DH 1) and Dagukong (EX-DH 20) acupoints on dorsal side of the hand; and digit-pressing Daling (PC 7) acupoint on palmar side of the hand and stomach holographic point on dorsal side of the hand.

2) Digit-pressing Dadu (SP 2), Gongsun (SP 4) and Taibai (SP 3) acupoints on the foot.

3) Rubbing heavily central part of palm and pushing dorsal interosseous spaces.

4) Rubbing heavily midline, medial and lateral borders of the sole; digit-pressing stomach, digestive tract, ear (balance organs) and head reflecting areas on the foot.

5) An acute attack should be treated by strong stimulation, and other acupoints and reflecting areas on the hand and foot also may be selected for use.

18. Diarrhea

Diarrhea is a common symptom of digestive diseases with symptoms such as increased bowel movement, loose or watery stool or feces with pus and blood, increased bowel gurgitation, abdominal pain, reduced food intake, fatigue, and dehydration.

Acupoints and reflecting areas: As shown in Fig. 5-18a and 5-18b.

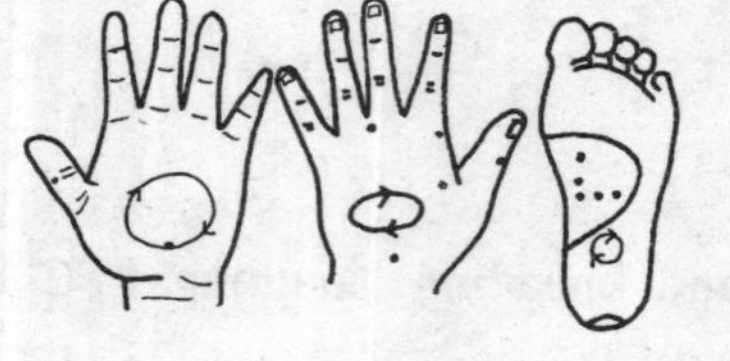

Fig. 5-18a

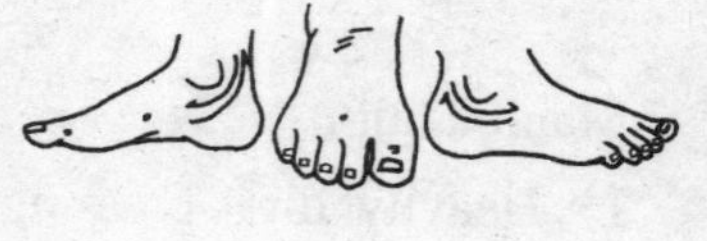

Fig. 5-18b

Manipulation:

1) Pressing and kneading chest pain (EX-PH 4) and stomach and intestine pain (EX-PH 8) acupoints on palmar side of the hand and Sanjian (LI 3), diarrhea (EX-PH 18), Yiwofeng (EX-PH 19) and Dagukong (EX-PH 20) acupoints and stomach holographic point on dorsal side of the hand.

2) Pressing and kneading No. 6 (EX-PF 9), No. 9 (EX-PF 12), colon (EX-PF 22), small intestine (EX-PF 24) and stomach (EX-PF 23) acupoints on plantar side of the foot

and Neiting (ST 44), Dadu (SP 2) and Gongsun (SP 4) acupoints on dorsal side of the foot.

3) Digit-pressing and kneading stomach, digestive tract, intestine and anus reflecting areas on the hand.

4) Digit-pressing and kneading stomach, digestive tract, intestine and anus reflecting areas on the foot; rubbing midline of the sole, and lateral and medial borders of malleolus.

5) Other acupoints and reflecting areas may also be selected for use. The quick and heavy manipulation is applied for acute cases; and the continuous and gentle manipulation for chronic cases. The Le'an No. 4 recipe is useful for foot bath.

19. Constipation

Constipation is delayed defecation due to impairment of bowel transmission. Symptoms include difficult voiding feces for prolonged intervals, although the patient has the desire to defecate. It is most common in sedentary people and the elderly.

Acupoints and reflecting areas: As shown in Fig. 5-19a and 5-19b.

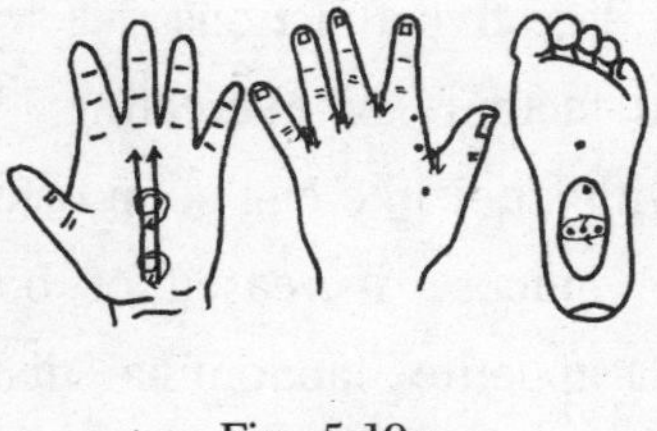

Fig. 5-19a

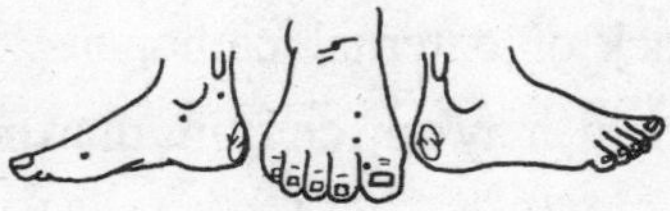

Fig. 5-19b

Manipulation:

1) Digit-pressing and kneading Erjian (LI 2), Sanjian (LI 3) and Hegu (LI 4) acupoints on dorsal side of the hand.

2) Pressing and kneading Yongquan (KI 1) acupoint on plantar side of the foot and Jiexi (ST 41), Taibai (SP 3), Dadun (LR 1), Xingjian (LR 2), Zhaohai (KI 6) and Dazhong (KI 4) acupoints on dorsal side of the foot; and kneading 3 Ludi acupoints (EX-PF 25) on plantar side of the foot.

3) Grinding and pushing intestine, anus and digestive tract reflecting areas on the hand; kneading the web borders between fingers.

4) Pushing intestine and anus reflecting areas on the foot; and kidney, urinary bladder and ureter holographic areas may be added for aged patients.

5) The Le'an No. 3 recipe may be used for hand and foot bath. Pressing head and adrenal gland holographic areas for severe cases; and gentle and continuous manipulation for senile constipation.

20. Indigestion

This is an impairment of the digestive functions due to an attack of external pathogens, food factors, or overeating. The patient may suffer from diarrhea with stool like egg soup or containing undigested food and some mucus, increased of bowel gurgitation, abdominal pain, poor appetite, abdominal distension and general weakness.

Acupoints and reflecting areas: As shown in Fig. 5-20a

and 5-20b.

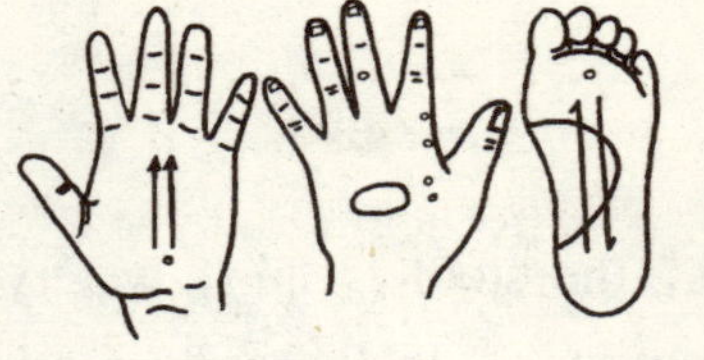

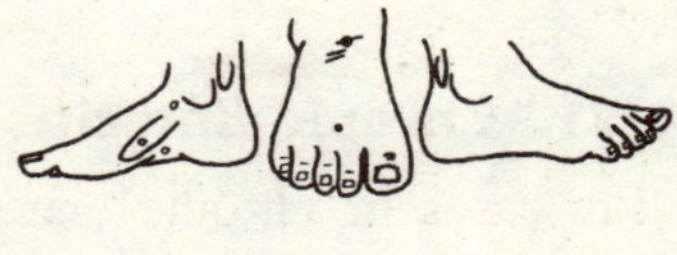

Fig. 5-20a   Fig. 5-20b

Manipulation:

1) Pressing and kneading stomach and intestine pain acupoint (EX-PH 8) on palmar side of the hand and Erjian (LI 2), Sanjian (LI 3) and Zhongkui (EX-DH 1) acupoints, and stomach and duodenum holographic points on dorsal side of the hand.

2) Digit-pressing and kneading Lineiting (EX-PF 2) acupoint on plantar side of the foot and Jiexi (ST 41), Neiting (ST 44) and Gongsun (SP 4) acupoints on dorsal side of the foot; and kneading Shangqiu (SP 5) and Rangu (KI 2) acupoints on dorsal side of the foot.

3) Grinding and pushing stomach, digestive tract, intestine, and pancreas holographic areas on the hand.

4) Pushing and pressing stomach, digestive tract and intestine holographic areas on the foot; and rubbing midline of the sole.

5) The Le'an No. 3 recipe can be used for foot bath before manipulation. The manipulation should be moderately or gently and persistently applied for a longer time. The correspondent

acupoints and areas may be added for indigestion caused by external pathogens.

21. Chronic Enteritis

In cases of chronic enteritis, the stool is thin, watery or mixed with a white gelatinous substance. In the early morning the patient usually has abdominal pain before diarrhea, and the discomfort may disappear right after bowel movement.

Acupoints and reflecting areas: As shown in Fig. 5-21a and 5-21b.

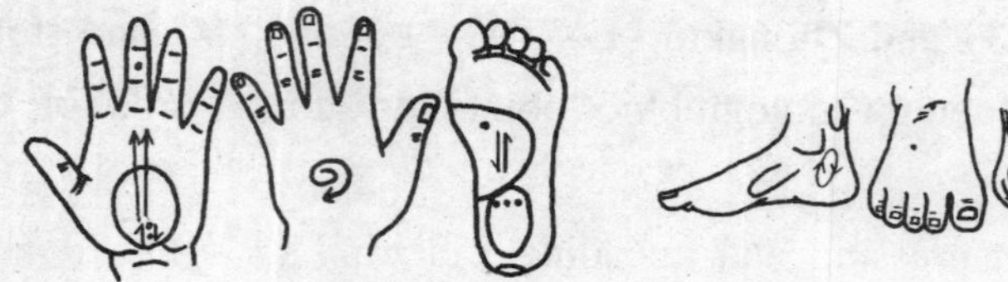

Fig. 5-21a   Fig. 5-21b

Manipulation:

1) Pinching and digit-pressing pelvic cavity (EX-PH 22), Banmen (EX-PH 27) and stomach and intestine pain (EX-PH 8) acupoints on palmar side of the hand.

2) Pressing and kneading pain-controlling (EX-PF 30) and 3 Ludi (EX-PF 35) acupoints on plantar side of the foot and Jiexi (ST 41) and No. 19 (EX-DF 10) on dorsal side of the foot; or digit-pressing No. 10 (EX-PF 13) acupoint on plantar side of the foot.

3) Grinding and pushing midline of palm, stomach and in-

testine, and kidney holographic areas of the hand; and rubbing proximal part of the palm.

4) Pushing and pressing stomach, intestine, urinary bladder, kidney and anus holographic areas on the foot; and rubbing heavily midline of the sole.

5) The Le'an No. 4 recipe may be used for hand and foot bath. The manipulation should be gently applied. In addition, the patient should follow a diet arranged by the practitioner.

22. Viral Hepatitis

Viral hepatitis is caused by a hepatitis virus infection and the patient may suffer from short-lived fever, general fatigue, poor appetite, nausea, abdominal distension, dull pain in liver region, and jaundice in some cases.

Acupoints and reflecting areas: As shown in Fig. 5-22a and 5-22b.

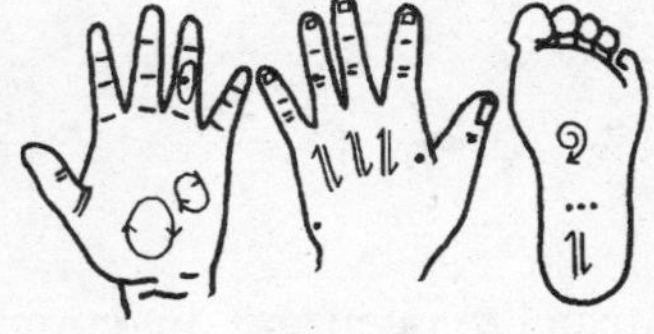

Fig. 5-22a

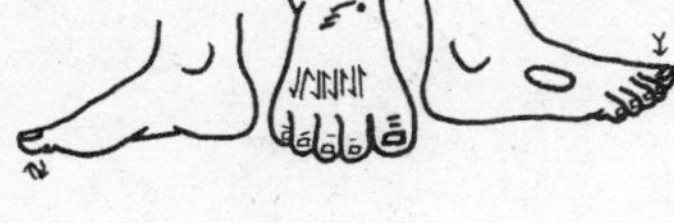

Fig. 5-22b

Manipulation:

1) Pinching and digit-pressing liver acupoint (EX-PH 21) on palmar side of the hand, Wangu (SI 4) and temporal headache (EX-DH 6c) acupoints and liver holographic point on

dorsal side of the hand.

2) Digit-pressing and kneading 3 Ludi acupoints (EX-PF 35) on plantar side of the foot and Zhongfeng (LR 4) acupoint on dorsal side of the foot.

3) Heavily kneading liver, gallbladder, stomach and kidney holographic areas on the hand; pushing and rubbing palm and dorsal interosseous spaces between metacarpal bones.

4) Digit-pressing liver and gallbladder holographic areas and grinding stomach and kidney holographic areas on the foot; heavily rubbing the sole and dorsal interosseous spaces between metatarsal bones; and pinching and twisting all sides of the toe.

5) The Le'an No. 2 recipe may be used for foot bath before above manipulation. The strong stimulation is applied to the sensitive spots. The correspondent acupoints and reflecting areas should be added for jaundice, and the medium manipulation should be applied.

23. Dysentery

This is an infectious disease usually occuring in summer and autumn with symtoms of abdominal pain, tenesmus, passing stool with white pus and red blood, fever, anorexia, burning sensation in anus, and dark urine in short streams.

Acupoints and reflecting areas: As shown in Fig. 5-23a and 5-23b.

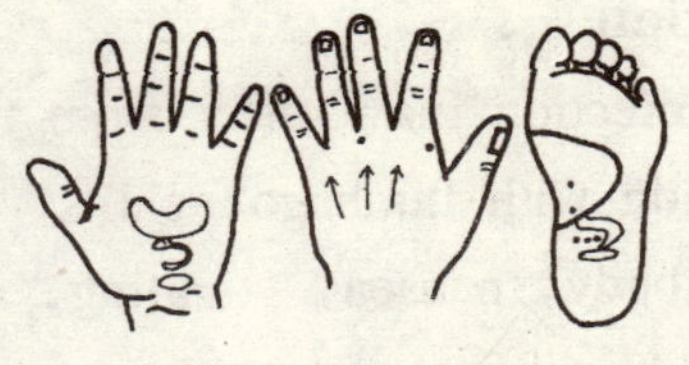 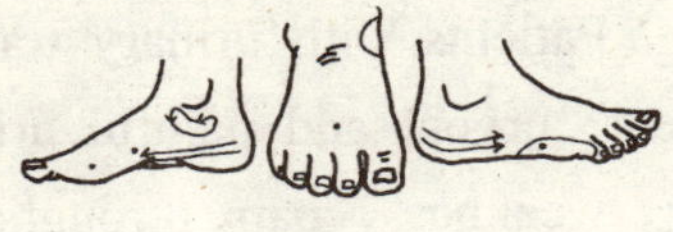

Fig. 5-23a   Fig. 5-23b

Manipulation:

1) Persistently digit-pressing and kneading Sanjian (LI 3) and diarrhea (EX-DH 18) acupoints on dorsal side of the hand.

2) Continuously digit-pressing No. 6 (EX-PF 9), No. 9 (EX-PF 12) and 3 Ludi (EX-PF 35) acupoints on plantar side of the foot; and Neiting (ST 44), Taibai (SP 3), Gongsun (SP 4) and Sugu (BL 65) acupoints on dorsal side of the foot.

3) Pressing and kneading stomach, intestine, urinary bladder and kidney reflecting areas on the hand; and pushing interosseous spaces between metacarpal bones on dorsum of the the hand.

4) Pressing and kneading stomach, intestine, related lymphatic, urinary bladder and kidney reflecting areas on the foot, and from midpoint of the heel along medial and lateral borders of the sole to tips of the big and little toes.

5) The Le'an No. 2 recipe or clean water may be used for foot bath. Other reflecting areas and related acupoints can be selected for use according to the disease, and the medium stimulation is best applied continously.

24. Urinary Tract Infection

Patients with urinary tract infection may suffer from frequent, urgent and painful urination with lumbago, chills, fever, weakness, pain throughout body, nausea, vomiting, abdominal distension, and turbid or bloody urine.

Acupoints and reflecting areas: As shown in Fig. 5-24a and 5-24b.

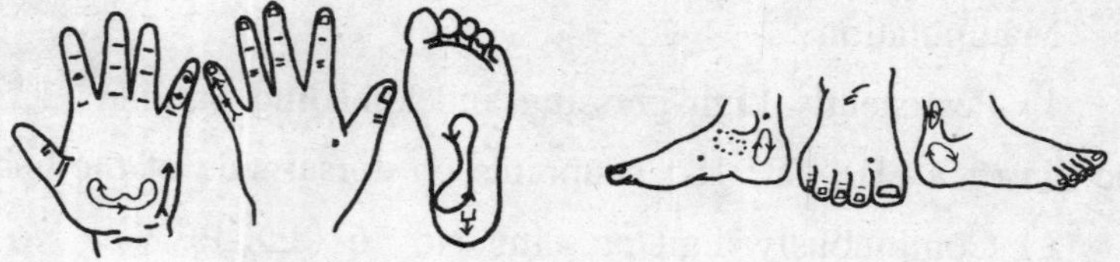

Fig. 5-24a   Fig. 5-24b

Manipulation:

1) Pinching and digit-pressing bed-wetting (EX-PH 12), urethra (EX-PH 15) and Mingmen (EX-PH 20) acupoints on palmar side of the hand; and lower abdomen holographic point on dorsal side of the hand.

2) Digit-pressing and kneading Xingjian (LR 2), Taixi (KI 3) and Gongsun (SP 4) acupoints on the foot.

3) Heavily kneading kidney and urinary bladder holographic areas on the hand; and pinching and kneading all sides of the little finger and ulnar half of the palm.

4) Digit-pressing kidney, urinary bladder and reproduction reflecting areas on the foot; stepping on heel and central part of the sole; and rubbing midline of the sole.

5) The Le'an No. 2 recipe may be used for foot bath before applying above manipulation. The manipulation should be forcibly applied to the deep tissues. Greater manipulation should be applied to the reflecting areas of the urogenital system.

25. Chronic Glomerulonephritis

Glomerulonephritis is an immune inflammatory disease of the glomeruli caused by many pathogenic factors. In mild cases, the edema appears only on the eyelids and ankle joints; but in severe cases it occurs all over the body causing soreness and pain of the waist, oligouria, loose stool, and weakness.

Acupoints and reflecting areas: As shown in Fig. 5-25a and 5-25b.

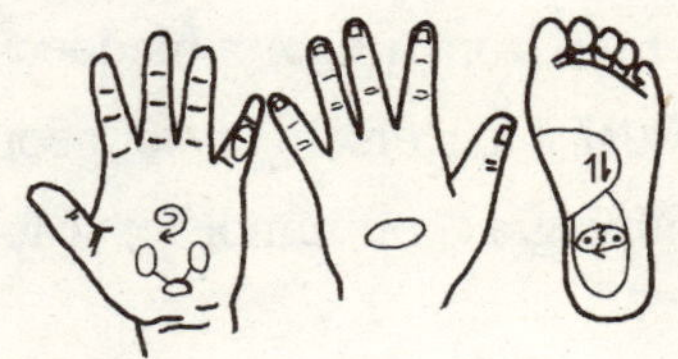

Fig. 5-25a   Fig. 5-25b

Manipulation:

1) Continuously digit-pressing and kneading 3 Ludi acupoints (EX-PF 35) on plantar side of the foot; and Jiexi (ST 41), Xian'gu (ST 43), Taibai (SP 3) and Taixi (KI 3) acupoints on dorsal side of the foot.

2) Persistently pressing and kneading kidney, ureter, urinary bladder, stomach and intestine reflecting areas on the

hand; and grinding central part of the palm.

3) Digit-pressing kidney, ureter, urinary bladder, stomach and intestine reflecting areas on the foot; pushing and rubbing central part of the sole; and pushing areas around medial and lateral malleoli.

4) The Le'an No. 2 and No. 4 recipes are used for foot bath before applying above manipulation. The manipulation should be continuously applied with a proper force and greater manipulation applied to the sensitive spots. The waist and kidney holographic areas may also be selected for use according to the disease.

26. Incontinence of Urine

The automatic discharge of urine from urinary bladder or uncontrollable dripping of urine usually occurs in aged people and patients with paraplegia, hemiplegia, or tumor of cauda equina.

Acupoints and reflecting areas: As shown in Fig. 5-26a and 5-26b.

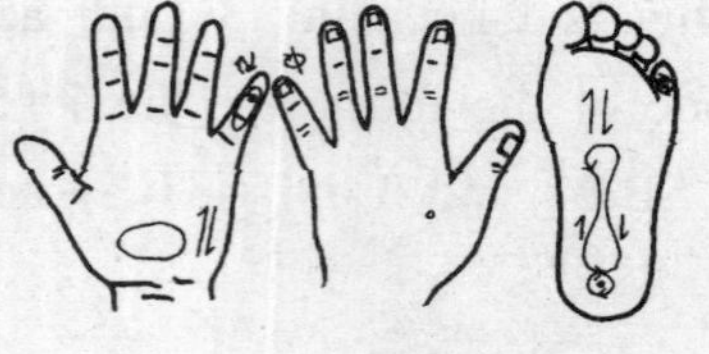

Fig. 5-26a

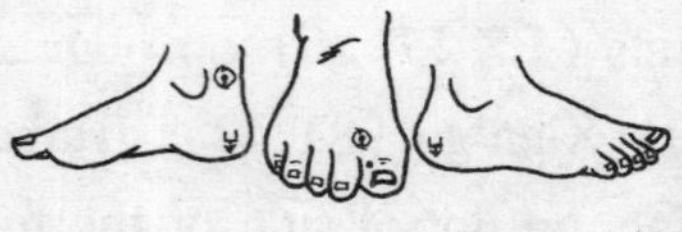

Fig. 5-26b

Manipulation:

1) Persistently pinching and kneading bed-wetting acupoint (EX-PH 12) on palmar side of the hand.

2) Continuously pressing and kneading Sibai acupoint at heel (EX-PF 42) and No. 14 acupoint (EX-PF 17) on plantar side of the foot, and Taixi (KI 3), Dadun (LR 10) and Xingjian (LR 2) acupoints on dorsal side of the foot.

3) Rubbing hypothenar prominence; twisting and kneading little finger; and pressing kidney and urinary bladder holographic areas on the hand.

4) Heavily rubbing sole; digit-pressing kidney, ureter and urinary bladder holographic areas on the foot; and stepping on heel.

5) The Le'an No. 1 and No. 4 recipes may be used for hand and foot bath before applying above manipulation. The manipulation should be continuously and gently applied until producing a local warmth which should be maintained. Other acupoints and reflecting areas may be selected according to the disease.

27. Prostatitis

Inflammation of the prostatic gland is caused by an infection of bacteria invading from nearby structures, and the patient may suffer from urgent, frequent, difficult and painful urination and dripping of urine, white and turbid urine like rice water, mental fatigue and attack of cold to waist and knee.

Acupoints and reflecting areas: As shown in Fig. 5-27a and 5-27b.

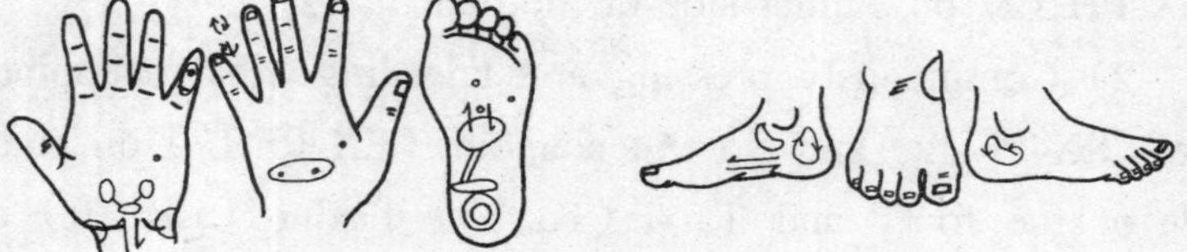

Fig. 5-27a   Fig. 5-27b

Manipulation:

1) Pinching and digit-pressing bed-wetting (EX-PH 12) and Shaofu (HT 8) acupoints on palmar side of the hand; and 2 waist and leg pain acupoints (EX-DH 3) and lower abdomen holographic point on dorsal side of the hand.

2) Kneading and pressing Yongquan (KI 1) and kidney (EX-PF 33) and urinary bladder (EX-PF 31) acupoints on plantar side of the foot.

3) Persistently pushing and pressing kidney, urinary bladder and other urogenital reflecting areas on the hand; rubbing proximal part of the palm; and twisting and rotating the little finger.

4) Continuously pushing and pressing areas of kidney, urinary bladder, reproduction and other areas of urogenital and related lymphatic organs; and rubbing and moving central part of the sole and medial side of the foot.

5) The Le'an No. 2 and No. 3 recipes are used for foot bath before applying above manipulation. The manipulation

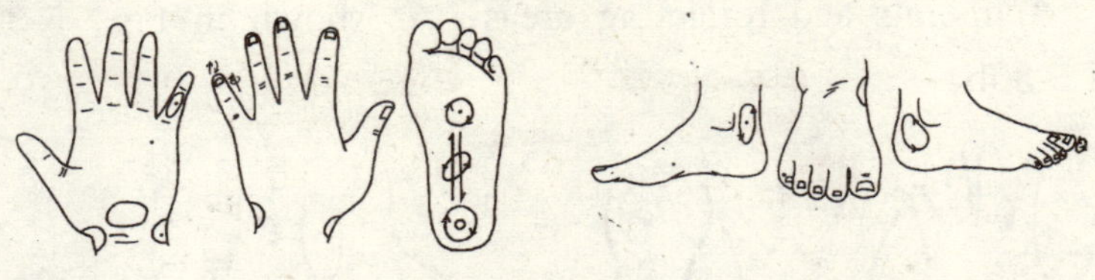

Fig. 5-29a   Fig. 5-29b

on plantar side of the foot and Taixi (KI 3), Gongsun (SP 4) and Zhiyin (BL 67) acupoints on dorsal side of the foot.

3) Continuously pressing and kneading kidney, reproduction and reproductive gland reflecting areas on the hand; and twisting and rotating the little finger.

4) Pressing and kneading reproduction and kidney holographic areas on the foot; pinching and kneading the big toe; and rubbing midline of the sole.

5) The Le'an No. 1 recipe is used for foot bath. The head and neurasthenia holographic areas and points, also may be selected in for use.

30. Facial Palsy

This is a disease with a sudden onset of stiffness, numbness and paralysis on one side of face in the morning after waking. The patient may also suffer from difficulty using facial muscles, deviation of the corner of the mouth to the healthy side, and dripping of saliva and lachrymation caused by blowing wind.

Acupoints and reflecting areas: As shown in Fig. 5-30a and 5-30b.

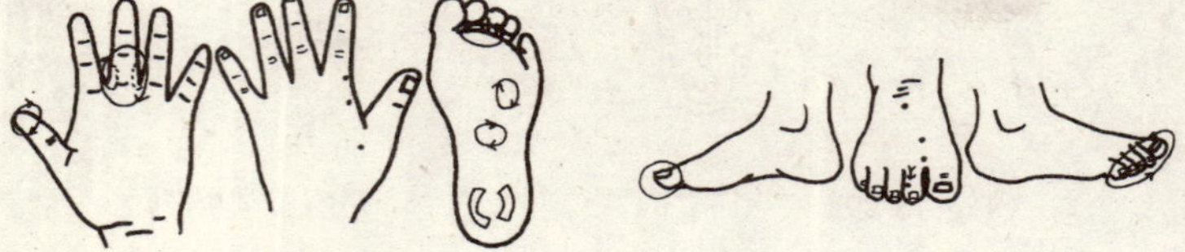

Fig. 5-30a   Fig. 5-30b

Manipulation:

1) Digit-pressing and kneading Erjian (LI 2) and Hegu (LI 4) acupoints, and head holographic area on dorsal side of the hand.

2) Digit-pressing and kneading Lidui (ST 45), Chongyang (ST 42), Xingjian (LR 2) and Taichong (LR 3) acupoints on the foot; or digit-pressing and pinching Lidui (ST 45).

3) Pressing and kneading head, mouth and eye reflecting areas on the hand; twisting, pulling, rotating and pinching all fingers.

4) Pressing and kneading head, mouth, eye, liver and kidney reflecting areas on the foot.

5) The Le'an No. 1 and No. 2 recipes can be used for hand and foot bath before manipulation. Manipulation intensity may be gradually increased and then decreased.

31. Trigeminal Neuralgia

This is a disease of the trigeminal nerve with a sudden onset of short-lived severe pain on one side of face. The pain may be cutting, burning, chiselling or pricking in nature, and can be induced by speaking or yawning. This condition is more common in women.

Acupoints and reflecting areas: As shown in Fig. 5-31a and 5-31b.

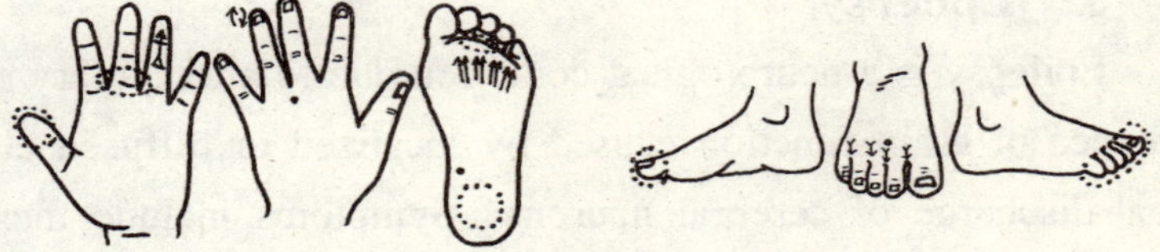

Fig. 5-31a   Fig. 5-31b

Manipulation:

1) Heavily pinching and digit-pressing sore throat acupoint (EX-DH 10) on dorsal side of the hand.

2) Heavily digit-pressing No. 2 acupoint (EX-PF 5) on plantar side of the foot and Neiting acupoint (ST 44) on dorsal side of the foot.

3) Heavily digit-pressing head, mouth and eye reflecting areas on the hand; and twisting and pinching different sides of the ring finger.

4) Heavily digit-pressing head, mouth and eye reflecting areas on the foot; pinching web borders of all toes; and heavily pushing interosseous spaces between metatarsal bones and meta-

tarsophalangeal joints on plantar side of the foot.

, 5) The strong stimulation may be applied during acute attack. The Le'an No. 1 and No. 3 recipes may be used for hand and foot bath after acute attacks. In general, the gentle and medium stimulation is applied and continued for adjustment of nervous system functions after the attack is controlled.

32. Epilepsy

Epilepsy is a neurological condition due to a temporary disturbance of brain function caused by localized or diffused electrical discharge of cerebral neurons. Symptoms include mental confusion, sudden falling, loss of consciousness, dilatation of pupils, saliva foaming from the mouth, upward staring, and convulsions of limbs.

Acupoints and reflecting areas: As shown in Fig. 5-32a and 5-32b.

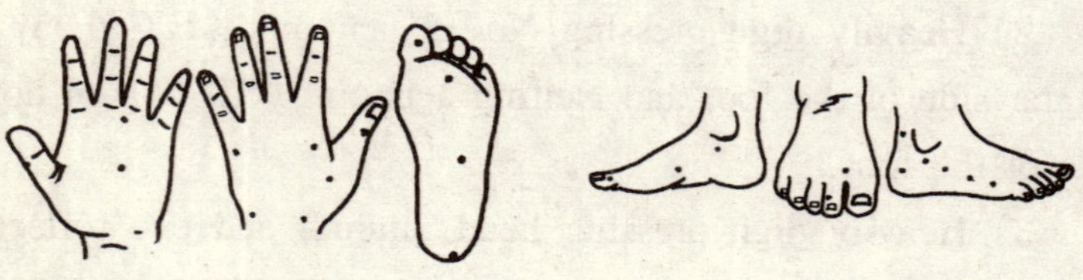

Fig. 5-32a   Fig. 5-32b

Manipulation:

1) Pinching and digit-pressing Shenmen (HT 7), Laogong

(PC 8), chest pain (EX-PH 4) and finger and palm (EX-PH 24) acupoints on palmar side of the hand; and Hegu (LI 4), Houxi (SI 3), Yanggu (SI 5), Shixuan (EX-PH 1), Bahui (EX-DH 24) and Hubian (EX-DH 32) acupoints on dorsal side of the hand.

2) Pinching and digit-pressing Lineiting (EX-PF 2), Nuxi (EX-PF 3) and No. 8 (EX-PF 11) acupoints on plantar side of the foot; and Jiexi (ST 41), Yinbai (SP 1), Gongsun (SP 4), Kunlun (BL 60), Jinmen (BL 63), Sugu (BL 65), Tonggu (BL 66), Pucan (BL 61), Zhaohai (KI 6), Shenmai (BL 62), Lidui (ST 45) and Xingjian (LR 2) acupoints on dorsal side of the foot.

3) Grind and pushing palm and dorsum of the hand and sole of the foot; twisting and rotating all fingers and toes; and especially pinching and pressing the big toe during the intervals between attacks.

4) Digit-pressing head holographic area and point with quick and strong stimulation during attacks.

33. Neurasthenia

Neurasthenia is usually caused by nervous tension and the patient may suffer from weakness, fatigue, high irritability, headache, insomnia, poor concentration, poor memmory, heart palpitations, cold limbs, loss of appetite, premature ejaculation of semen, impotence, or irregular menstruation.

Acupoints and reflecting areas: As shown in Fig. 5-33a and 5-33b.

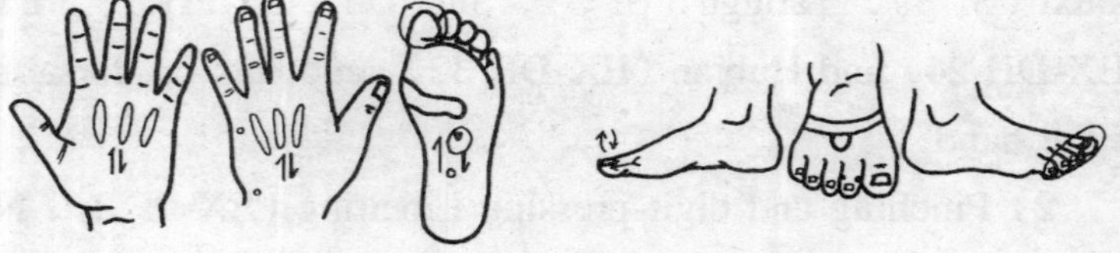

Fig. 5-33a   Fig. 5-33b

Manipulation:

1) Persistently pressing and kneading Shenmen (HT 7) acupoint on palmar side of the hand; and Houxi (SI 3), Shaoshang (LU 11) and Yanggu (SI 5) acupoints on dorsal side of the hand.

2) Continuously digit-pressing and kneading No. 8 (EX-PF 11) and No. 3 (EX-PF 6) acupoints on plantar side of the foot; and Qingtou 1 (EX-DF 26) and Lidui (ST 45) acupoints on dorsal side of the foot.

3) Pressing and kneading interosseous spaces between metacarpal bones on palmar and dorsal sides of the hand; rubbing dorsum of the hand.

4) Rubbing central part of the sole; twisting and pinching all toes; and pressing head, heart and kidney holographic areas on the foot.

5) The Le'an No. 1 recipe can be used for hand and foot bath before manipulation. The manipulation should be gently and continuously applied and other related acupoints and reflect-

ing areas can be selected for use according to the disease.

34. Hysteria

This is a disease more common in women with complicated symptoms, including convulsions, monoplegia, hemiplegia or paraplegia, and erratic behavior, such as madly shouting, chest beating and stamping feet, loudly singing and speaking nonsense at any time or place, or playing the fool, acting out, and being impolite to people of any age.

Acupoints and reflecting areas: As shown in Fig. 5-34a and 5-34b.

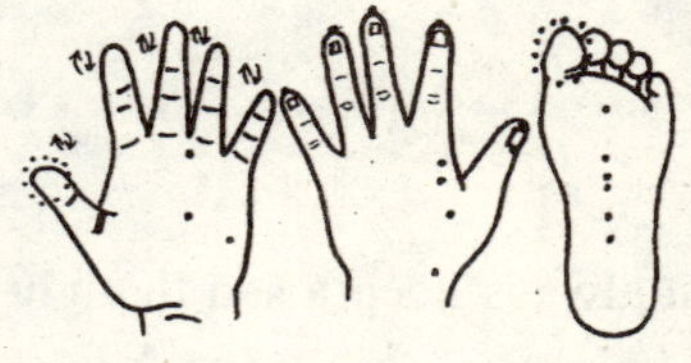

Fig. 5-34a   Fig. 5-34b

Manipulation:

1) Heavily pinching Laogong (PC 8) and hypothenar (EX-PH 23) acupoints on palmar side of the hand; and Shixuan (EX-PH 1), Hegu (LI 4), Shaoshang (LU 11), Baihui (EX-DH 24) and Hubian (EX-DH 32) acupoints on dorsal side of the hand; and digit-pressing finger and palm acupoint (EX-PH 24).

2) Heavily digit-pressing Yongquan (KI 1), No. 3 (EX-PF 6), Quan'gen (EX-PF 39), Quanzhong (EX-PF 40),

Quanding (EX-PF 41) and pericardium (EX-PF 26) acupoints on plantar side of the foot; and Pucan (BL 61), Tonggu (BL 66), Shangqiu (SP 5), Zhaohai (KI 6) and Qingtou 1 (EX-DF 26) acupoints on dorsal side of the foot.

3) Heavily pinching nail root of fingers and toes; twisting and pulling all fingers; and heavily digit-pressing head holographic area and point during attacks of hysteria.

4) The gentle or medium stimulation may be applied to above acupoints and reflecting areas during the intervals between attacks, and the intensity of stimulation may be gradually increased to elevate the tolerance of the patient and prevent relapse.

35. Mental Depression

People with mental depression always keep a sad thought in mind. They cannot correctly apprehend the world and everything in the world seems bad to them. They also may suffer from insomnia, sleepiness, weakness, irritability, and soreness and body pain without apparent cause.

Acupoints and reflecting areas: As shown in Fig. 5-35a

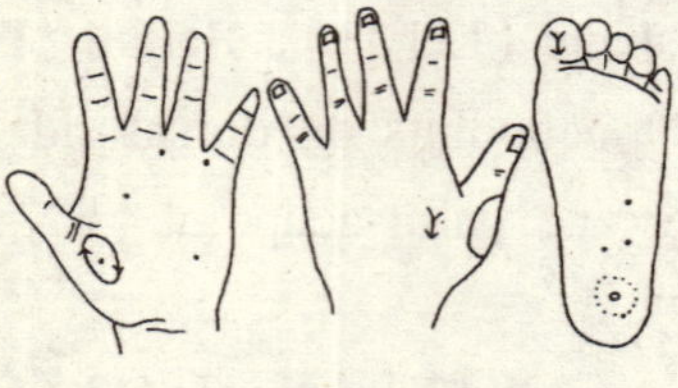

Fig. 5-35a 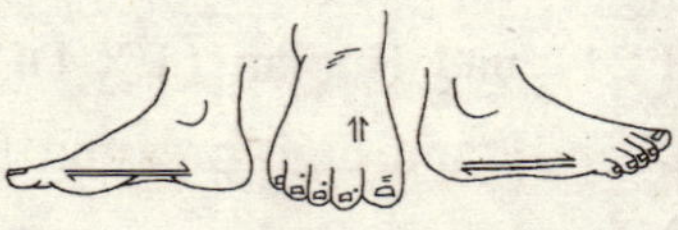   Fig. 5-35b

and 5-35b.

Manipulation:

1) Digit-pressing heart palpitation (EX-PH 13), finger and palm (EX-PH 24), Laogong (PC 8), hypothenar (EX-PH 23) and endocrine (EX-PH 3) acupoints on palmar side of the hand; and heavily pinching Hegu (LI 4) acupoint.

2) Persistently digit-pressing No. 3 (EX-PF 3), No. 8 (EX-PF 11), ear (EX-PF 21), Qingtou 1 (EX-DF 26), Qingtou 2 (EX-DF 27) and Qingtou 3 (EX-DF 28) acupoints on the foot; and heavily pinching plantar side of the big toe.

3) Persistently and gently pressing and kneading thenar prominence and endocrine holographic area on dorsal side of the thumb.

4) Deeply digit-pressing the heel; pushing space between 1st and 2nd metatarsal bones (liver meridian); and rubbing medial side of first metatarsal bone and lateral side of 5th metatarsal bone until a hot sensation is produced.

5) The Le'an No. 1 recipe can be used for foot bath. The acupoints and reflecting areas for adjusting liver and spleen and tranquilizing the mind can be selected for use, and psychotherapy should be utilized together with hand and foot massage.

36. Hyperthyroidism

This is an endocrinal disease due to an over excretion of the thyroid hormone caused by many pathogenic factors. The patient may suffer from mental nervousness, emotional disturbance, heart palpitations, tachycardia, weight loss, exophthalmus, and increased bowel movement.

Acupoints and reflecting areas: As shown in Fig. 5-36a and Fig. 5-36b.

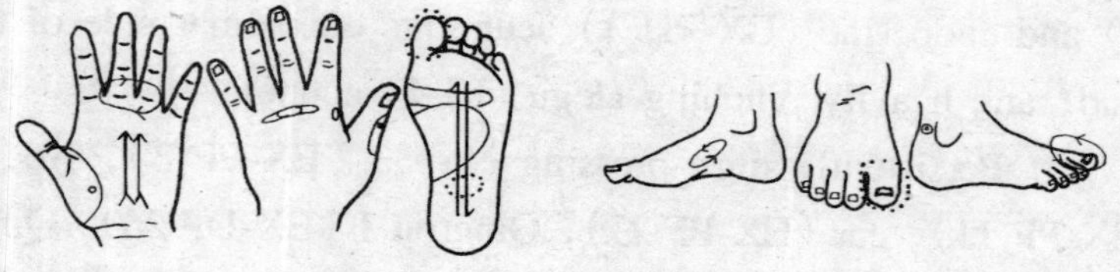

Fig. 5-36a   Fig. 5-36b

1) Persistently kneading and pressing endocrine acupoint (EX-PH 3) on palmar side of the hand; and head and neck holographic points on dorsal side of the hand.

2) Continuously digit-pressing Kunlun (BL 60) acupoint on dorsal side of the foot.

3) Persistently pressing and kneading head, neck, heart, eye, intestine and stomach reflecting areas on the hand; and pinching and pushing midline of palm from proximal end of the middle finger.

4) Heavily digit-pressing neck, thyroid gland, heart, stomach and intestine holographic areas on the foot; and heavily rubbing midline of the sole.

5) The Le'an No. 3 recipe can be used for hand and foot bath. Other appropriate acupoints and reflecting areas may be selected for use, and the manipulation should be moderately and continuously applied. Daily life and diet should be properly ar-

ranged under supervision of the practitioner.

37. Rheumatoid Arthritis

Rheumatoid arthritis is a generalized disease of the peripheral small joints with symmetrical lesions on the hand, wrist and
foot. Symptoms in the early stages are redness, swelling, hotness, pain and limitation of movement of involved joints; and
symptoms in the late stages include stiffness and deformity of
the joints.

Acupoints and reflecting areas: As shown in Fig. 5-37a
and 5-37b.

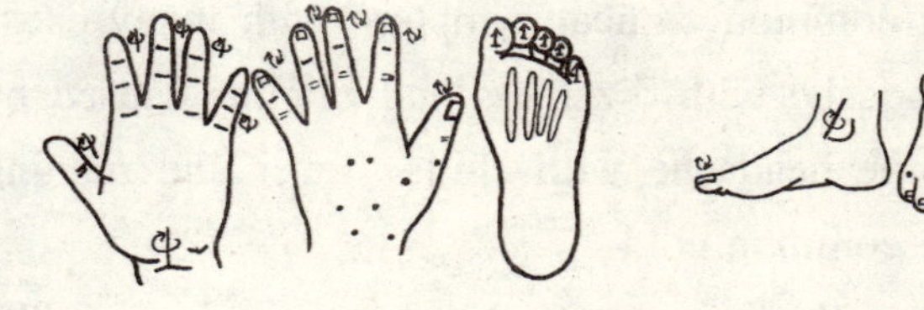

Fig. 5-37a   Fig. 5-37b

Manipulation:

1) Digit-pressing and kneading Hegu (LI 4), Yangxi (LI
5), waist and leg pain (EX-DH 3), Wailaogong (EX-DH 22),
Yinmen (EX-DH 33), Hujincun (EX-DH 40) and frontal headache (EX-DH 6a) acupoints on dorsal side of the hand.

2) Digit-pressing and kneading Zhiping (EX-DF 5) and
Diwuhui (GB 42) acupoints on dorsal side of the foot.

3) Pressing and kneading all small joints of the hand to
wrist joint; heavily pressing dorsal interosseous spaces; and

twisting, pulling and rotating all fingers and wrist joint.

4) Pressing and kneading all small joints of the foot to ankle joint; heavily pressing or pushing dorsal and plantar interosseous spaces; and twisting, pulling and rotating all toes and ankle joint.

5) The Le'an No. 1 recipe can be used for hand and foot bath before manipulation. Other acupoints and reflecting areas can be selected for use for other symptoms, and the manipulation should be gently and nimbly applied.

38. Headache

Headache is a common clinical symptom with many causes, such as the headache with dizziness and tinnitus caused by hypertension, and the headache with chills, fever and running nose caused by the common cold.

Acupoints and reflecting areas: As shown in Fig. 5-38a and 5-38b.

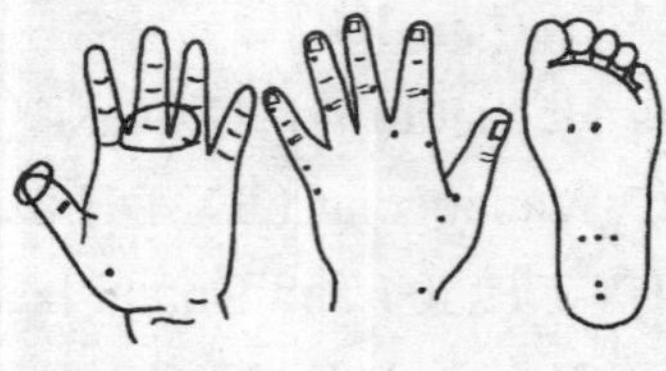

Fig. 5-38a   Fig. 5-38b

Manipulation:

1) Pinching and digit-pressing Yuji (LU 10) on palmar side of the hand; and Hegu (LI 4), Yangxi (LI 5), Shaoze

(SI 1), Qian'gu (SI 2), Houxi (SI 3), Guanchong (TE 1), Headache (EX-DH 6), brain (EX-DH 14) and head holographic point on dorsal side of the hand.

2) Digit-pressing and kneading 3 Ludi (EX-PF 35), No. 1 (EX-PF 4), head (EX-PF 20), liver (EX-PF 32), kidney (EX-PF 33) and Sibai at heel (EX-PF 42) acupoints on plantar side of the foot; and Qingtou 1 (EX-DF 26), Qingtou 2 (EX-DF 27), Zhiyin (BL 67), Jiexi (ST 41), Shenmai (BL 62), Jinggu (BL 64), Lidui (ST 45), Zhaohai (KI 6), Xingjian (LR 2), Taichong (LR 3), Taixi (KI 3), Xiaxi (GB 43), No. 24 to No. 26 (EX-DF 15-17), No. 30 (EX-DF 21), Kunlun (BL 60) and Tonggu (BL 66) acupoints on dorsal side of the foot.

3) Digit-pressing head reflecting area on the hand and foot during and between attacks. Other acupoints and reflecting areas can also be selected for use, such as acupoints and reflecting areas to strengthen the kidney for headaches due to kidney deficiency. During an attack of headache, the strong stimulation should be applied.

39. Low Fever

Low fever usually occurs in postpartum and postoperative patients or those after childbrith or operation, or with chronic lingering diseases. The patient may suffer from on and off fever, dizziness, mental fatigue, spontaneous or night sweating, hotness in palm and sole, or some subjective feverishness without elevated body temperature.

Acupoints and reflecting areas: As shown in Fig. 5-39a and 5-39b.

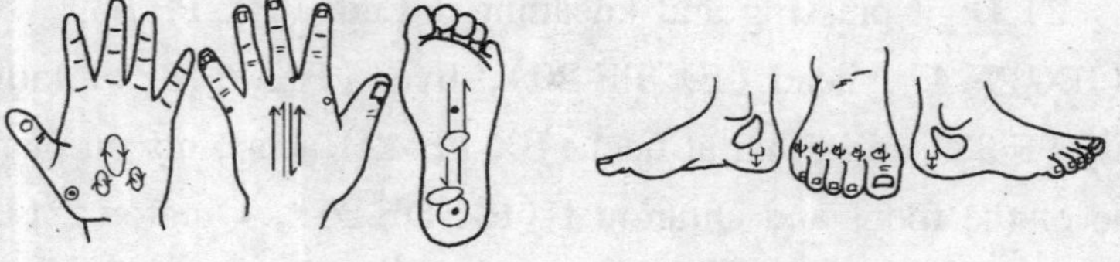

Fig. 5-39a   Fig. 5-39b

Manipulation:

1) Pressing and kneading Yuji (LU 10) acupoint on palmar side of the hand; and antifebrile acupoint (EX-DH 43), Shaoshang (LU 11), Shaochong (HT 9), Sanjian (LI 3), Shaoze (SI 1) and Qian'gu (SI 2) acupoints on dorsal side of the hand.

2) Digit-pressing and kneading Yongquan (KI 1) and insomnia (EX-PF 1) acupoints on plantar side of the foot.

3) Pressing and kneading head, stomach and intestine, and kidney reflecting areas on the hand; and pushing and rubbing dorsal, radial and ulnar sides of the 3rd metacarpal bone.

4) Pressing and kneading urinary bladder, kidney and reproduction holographic areas on the foot; rotating and twisting all toes, rubbing midline of the sole and stepping on the sole.

5) The Le'an No. 1, No. 2, No. 3 or No. 4 recipes may be used for hand and foot bath before carrying out above manipulation. Other symptomatic acupoints and reflecting areas may

also be selected for use, and the manipulation should be performed gently and persistently for a long time to produce a local
redness and hotness.

40. Menstrual Disorder

The disturbance of the menstrual period is called menstrual
disorder. It is called early menstrual cycle if the menstrual flow
starts 7 days before the regular cycle or comes twice a month; it
is called delayed menstrual cycle, if the menstrual flow is post-
poned for 7 days or even as much as 40 to 50 days; and it is
called irregular menstrual cycle if the menstrual flow comes irregularly, either early or delayed for over 7 days from time to time.

Acupoints and reflecting areas: As shown in Fig. 5-40a
and 5-40b.

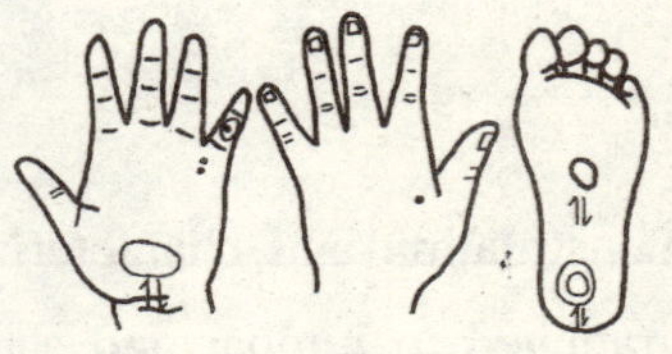

Fig. 5-40a   Fig. 5-40b

Manipulation:

1) Digit-pressing and kneading uterus (EX-PH 5), Mingmen (EX-PH 20) and heart palpitation (EX-PH 13) acupoints
on palmar side of the hand; and lower abdomen holographic
point on dorsal side of the hand.

2) Digit-pressing and kneading Bafeng (EX-DF 3), Taixi

(KI 3), Xingjian (LR 2), Zhaohai (KI 6), Gongsun (SP 4), Ran'gu (KI 2) and Shuiquan (KI 5) acupoints on the foot.

3) Persistently pressing and kneading reproduction and kidney holographic areas on the hand; and rubbing proximal part of the palm.

4) Continuously pressing and kneading reproduction and reproductive gland holographic areas in women, and kidney area on the foot; and rubbing central part of the sole and heel.

5) The Le'an No. 1 recipe can be used for foot bath before above manipulation. The manipulation should be applied moderately and persistently. Patients with prolonged menstrual disorder should receive further examinations to rule out serious organic lesions.

41. Dysmenorrhea

This is a disease related to menstruation and characterized by periodic lower abdominal pain radiated to lumbar and sacral region, and causing fainting in cases of severe pain. The attack may appear before, during, or after menstrual discharge, accompanied by scanty menstruation, obstructed menstruation mixed with dark purple clots, and weakness of waist and knee. It is most common in young women.

Acupoints and reflecting areas: As shown in Fig. 5-41a and 5-41b.

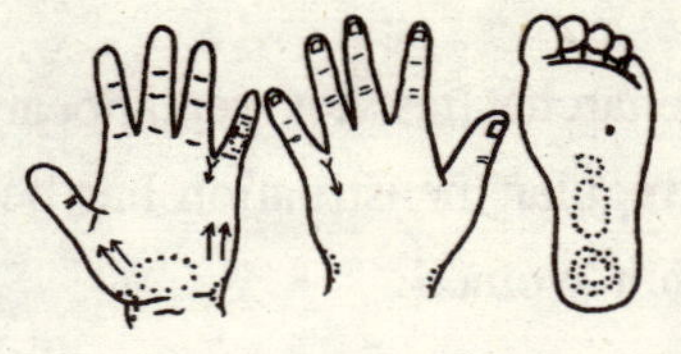 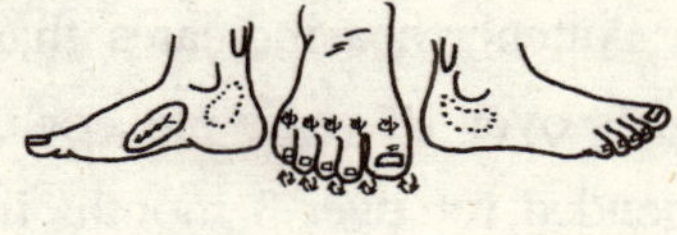

Fig. 5-41a   Fig. 5-41b

Manipulation:

1) Heavily pinching uterus (EX-PH 5) and heart palpitation (EX-PH 13) acupoints on palmar side of the hand.

2) Pinching and digit-pressing pain-controlling acupoint (EX-PF 30) on plantar side of the foot; and Gongsun (SP 4) and No. 28 (EX-PF 19) acupoints on dorsal side of the foot.

3) Heavily digit-pressing kidney, reproduction and reproductive gland reflecting areas on the hand; pushing thenar and hypothenar prominences; and pinching and pressing interosseous space between 4th and 5th metacarpal bones.

4) Heavily digit-pressing reproduction, reproductive gland, kidney and abdomen reflecting areas on the foot; heavily digit-pressing the heel; and twisting and rotating all toes.

5) The Le'an No. 1 recipe can be used for foot bath before applying above manipulation. The strong stimulation should be applied during an attack of dysmenorrhea, but the manipulation should be moderately applied thereafter to prevent dysmenorrhea and maintain health.

42. Amenorrhea

Amenorrhea indicates that menarche has not yet appeared in girls over 18 years old, or that regular menstruation has been suspended for over 3 months in adult women.

Acupoints and reflecting areas: As shown in Fig. 5-42a and 5-42b.

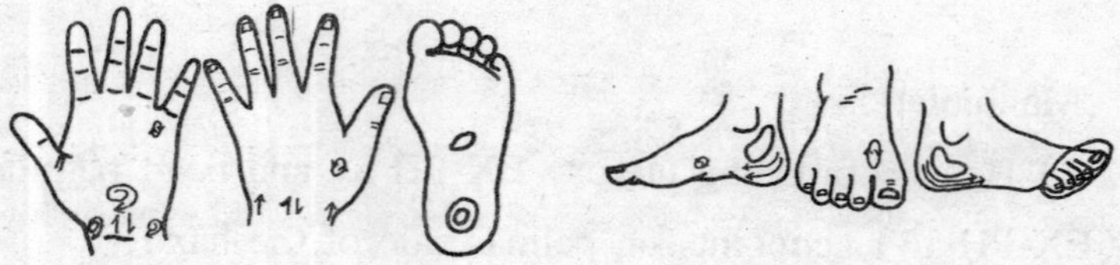

Fig. 5-42a   Fig. 5-42b

Manipulation:

1) Digit-pressing and kneading (combined with steaming and moxibustion) uterus (EX-PH 5) acupoint on palmar side of the hand, and Hegu (LI 4) acupoint on dorsal side of the hand.

2) Deeply digit-pressing and kneading Gongsun (SP 4) acupoint on dorsal side of the foot for a longer time.

3) Grinding and pushing reproduction and kidney reflecting areas on the hand; and rubbing dorsal and palmar sides of the wrist joint.

4) Heavily pressing reproduction, oviduct, ovary, kidney and head reflecting areas on the foot; and pushing bilateral borders of heel and instep of the foot with the intensity of manipulation gradually increased.

5) The Le'an No. 1 recipe can be used for foot bath before

applying above manipulation. The cause of amenorrhea should be found before starting hand and foot massage, and the manipulation should be continuous and medium in intensity. Other acupoints and reflecting areas also may be selected for use.

43. Functional Uterine Bleeding

This is a menstruation disorder usually appearing in the adolescent and menopausal stages with increased, prolonged and irregular menstrual discharge accompanied by dizziness, heart palpitations, insomnia, poor appetite, uncontollable fury, or high irritability.

Acupoints and reflecting areas: As shown in Fig. 5-43a and 5-43b.

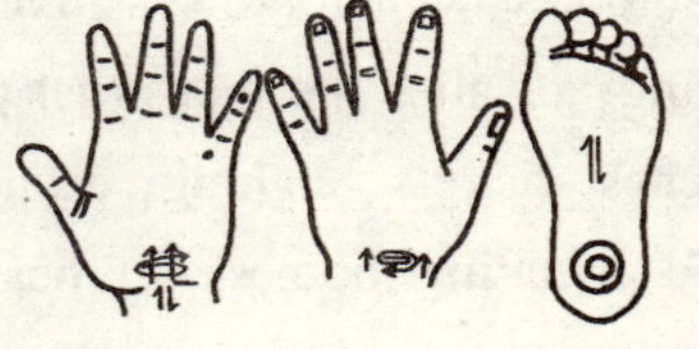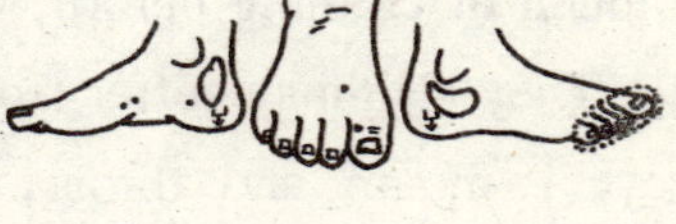

Fig. 5-43a   Fig. 5-43b

Manipulation:

1) Pinching and digit-pressing uterus (EX-PH 5) and bedwetting (EX-PH 12) acupoints on palmar side of hand.

2) Moderately digit-pressing and kneading No. 28 (EX-DF 19), No. 29 (EX-DF 20), Taichong (LR 3), Dadun (LR 1) and Gongsun (SP 4) acupoints on dorsal side of the foot.

3) Pushing and grinding reproduction holographic area on

the hand; and rubbing proximal part of the palm.

4) Digit-pressing head, reproduction, uterus and ovary holographic areas on the foot; stepping on the heel; and rubbing central part of the sole.

5) The Le'an No. 3 recipe may be used for foot bath before applying above manipulation. The acupoints and reflecting areas for heart palpitation and insomnia also may be selected for use. The manipulation can be applied with a gradually increased intensity, and then repeated several times. A gentle and proper manipulation can be applied after the profuse bleeding is controlled.

44. Menstrual Breast Distension and Pain

Patients with this condition suffer from breasts distension and swelling, itching and pain of nipples, which are sensitive to the touch of clothing before, during, or after the menstrual period. They also may suffer from chest distress, sighing, dryness in eyes, mouth and throat, and irritating hotness in heart, palms and soles.

Acupoints and reflecting areas: As shown in Fig. 5-44a and 5-44b.

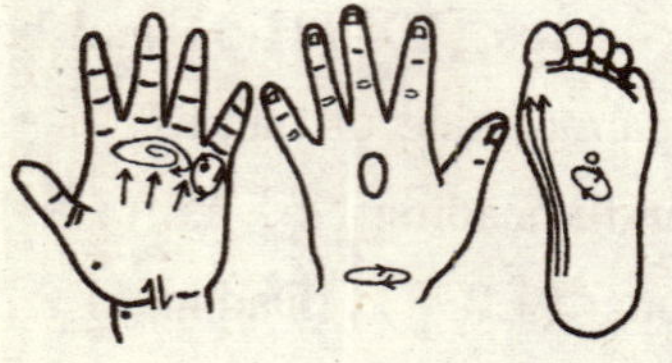

Fig. 5-44a

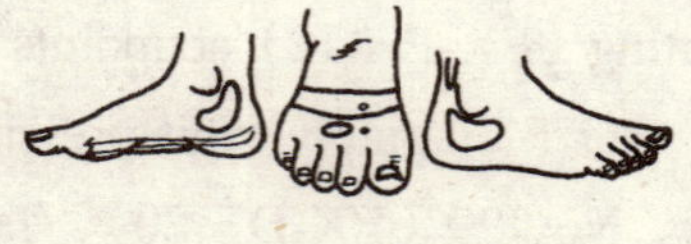

Fig. 5-44b

Manipulation:

1) Digit-pressing and kneading Taiyuan (LU 9), Yuji (LU 10) and uterus (EX-PH 5) acupoints on palmar side of the hand.

2) Digit-pressing Yongquan (KI 1) acupoint on plantar side of the foot; and Xingjian (LR 2) and Taichong (LR 3) acupoints on dorsal side of the foot.

3) Pushing metacarpophalangeal joints and interosseous spaces between metacarpal bones on palmar side of the hand; rubbing proximal part of the palm; and digit-pressing and kneading chest, lung, kidney and reproduction holographic areas on the hand.

4) Pressing and pushing chest, diaphragm, reproduction, ovary, uterus and kidney reflecting areas on the foot; and pushing spinal column holographic area on the foot.

5) The Le'an No. 1 recipe may be used for foot bath before applying above, manipulation and the foot bath warmth should be maintained. The acupoints and reflecting areas of head and chest may also be selected for use, combined with deep breathing and chest expansion exercises. The intensity of manipulation may be gradually increased and the range of exercise may also be gradually increased.

45. Menstrual Headache

Patients with this condition often suffer from headache before, during, or after the menstrual period accompanied by dizziness, vertigo, heart palpitations, weakness, pain in lower abdomen, bitter taste in mouth, and irritability.

Acupoints and reflecting areas: As shown in Fig. 5-45a and 5-45b.

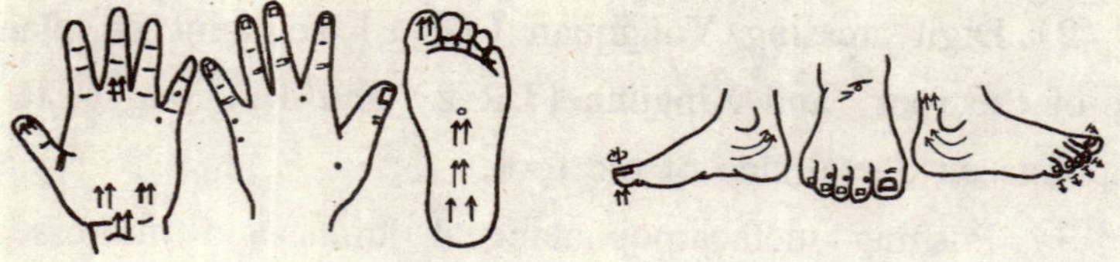

Fig. 5-45a   Fig. 5-45b

Manipulation:

1) Digit-pressing uterus (EX-PH 5) and Mingmen (EX-PH 20) acupoints on palmar side of the hand, and Hegu (LI 4), Shaoze (SI 1), Qian'gu (SI 2), Houxi (SI 3), Yemen (TE 2) and headache (EX-DH 6) acupoints on dorsal side of the hand.

2) Pressing and kneading Yongquan (KI 1) acupoint on plantar side of the foot; and Jiexi (ST 41) and No. 24 to No. 26 (EX-DF 15 to EX-DF 17) acupoints on dorsal side of the foot.

3) Pushing and grinding reproduction, kidney and head reflecting areas on the hand.

4) Heavily pushing reproduction, kidney, head and intestine reflecting areas on the foot; and rotating and pulling all toes.

5) The Le'an No. 3 recipe may be used for foot bath before applying above manipulation. The manipulation should be heavily and deeply applied during an attack of headache, but moderately thererafter. Other acupoints and reflecting areas for complications may also be selected in for use.

46. Menopausal Syndrome

This is a group of symptoms related to menopause in some of women which include vertigo, tinnitus, a hot feeling in body, sweating, heart palpitations, insomnia, irritability and anger, and hectic fever; or edema of face, eyes, and lower limbs, poor appetite, and loose stool; or menstrual disorder and mental instability.

Acupoints and reflecting areas: As shown in Fig. 5-46a and 5-46b.

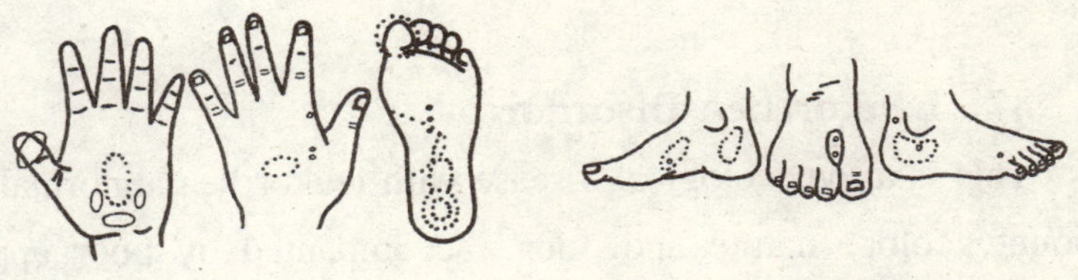

Fig. 5-46a   Fig. 5-46b

Manipulation:

1) Digit-pressing head, waist and kidney holographic points on dorsal side of the hand.

2) Digit-pressing Yongquan (KI 1), Quanzhong (EX-PF 40) and Quanding (EX-PF 41) acupoints on plantar side of the foot; and Taichong (LR 3), Xingjian (LR 2), Xiaxi (GB 43), Shenmai (BL 62), Kunlun (BL 60) and Gongsun (SP 4) acupoints on dorsal side of the foot.

3) Digit-pressing and kneading head, kidney, genital or-

gan, intestine and stomach reflecting areas on the hand.

4) Digit-pressing and kneading head (pituitary gland), reproduction, stomach, intestine and kidney reflecting areas on
the foot.

5) The Le'an No. 4 recipe can be used for foot bath before
applying above manipulation. Other acupoints and reflecting areas for various symptoms may be selected for use, and the manipulation should be moderately applied. Hand and foot massage
should be applied persistently in the morning and at night before
going to bed.

47. Leukorrhea Disorder

This is a gynecological disease with leukorrhea abnormal in
amount, color, nature and odor, accompanied by poor appetite, loose stool, and edema of feet; or soreness in waist and
long stream of clear urine; or abdominal pain and dry stool.
Leukorrhea disorder is divided into white, blue, and yellow leukorrhea in traditional Chinese medicine.

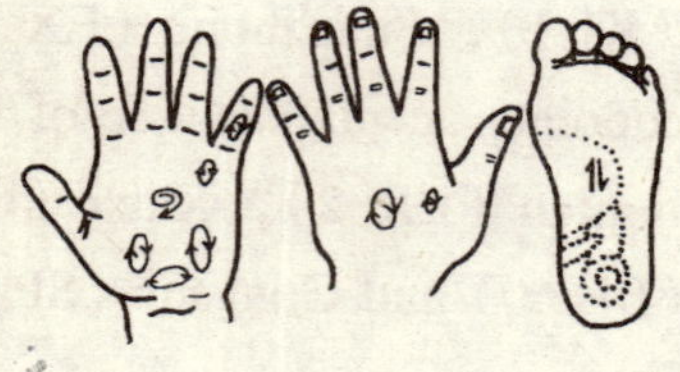

Fig. 5-47a

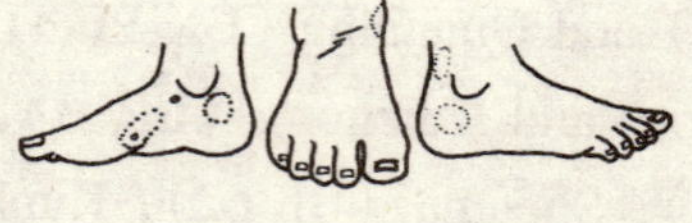

Fig. 5-47b

Acupoints and reflecting areas: As shown in Fig. 5-47a and 5-47b.

Manipulation:

1) Digit-pressing and kneading Mingmen (EX-PH 20) and uterus (EX-PH 5) acupoints on palmar side of the hand and lower abdomen holographic point on dorsal side of the hand.

2) Persistently digit-pressing Zhaohai (KI 6) and Gongsun (SP 4) acupoints on dorsal side of the foot.

3) Pressing and kneading kidney, reproduction, ovary, urinary bladder, stomach and intestine reflecting areas on the hand; and grinding central part of the palm.

4) Digit-pressing and kneading reproduction, ovary, uterus, urinary bladder, stomach and intestine reflecting areas of the foot; and heavily rubbing central part of the sole.

5) The Le'an No. 3 recipe may be used for foot bath. The manipulation should be continuously and moderately applied and other acupoints and reflecting areas for related symptoms may be selected for use.

48. Pregnancy Vomiting

In the early stage of pregnancy, the pregnant women may suffer from nausea and vomiting in the morning, along with dizziness, anorexia, or regurgitation of sour and bitter fluid, fullness and pain in chest and flank, belching and sighing, bitter taste in mouth, and irritability. These sympstoms may disappear in about 3 months.

Acupoints and reflecting areas: As shown in Fig. 5-48a and 5-48b.

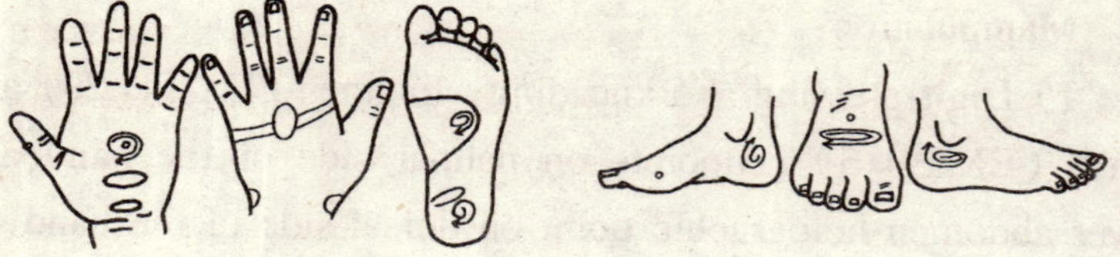

Fig. 5-48a   Fig. 5-48b

Manipulation:

1) Pressing and kneading Laogong (PC 8) and chest pain (EX-PH 4) acupoints on palmar side of the hand, and Zhongkui (EX-DH 1) and Dagukong (EX-DH 20) acupoints on dorsal side of the hand.

2) Pressing and kneading Chongyang (ST 42) and Taibai (SP 3) on acupoints on dorsal side of the foot.

3) Grinding and pressing stomach, chest, diaphragm and reproductive gland reflecting areas on the hand; and grinding central part of the palm to produce hotness.

4) Grinding and pressing stomach, chest, diaphragm, kidney, reproduction and urinary bladder holographic areas on the foot; and rubbing central part of the sole to produce hotness.

5) The Le'an No. 4 recipe or clean water may be used for foot bath. The manipulation should be applied continuously and gently, and the strong stimulation and sudden pressure increase should be avoided as this may have harmful effects on the fetus.

49. Threatened Abortion

A pregnant women with a threatened abortion may have a small amount of bloody discharge from vagina from time to time, accompanied by soreness in waist and abdominal pain or lower abdominal distension and strain.

Acupoints and reflecting areas: As shown in Fig. 5-49a and 5-49b.

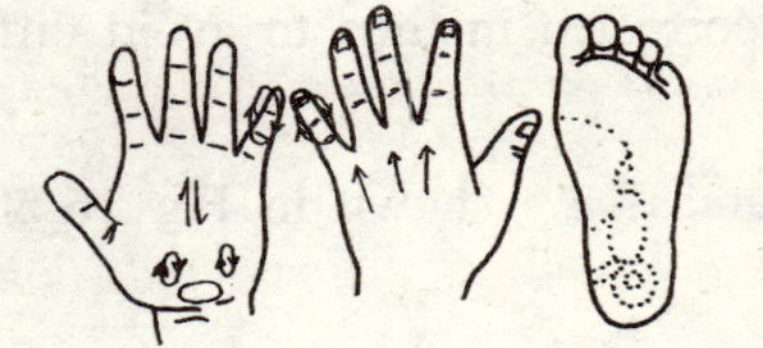

Fig. 5-49a

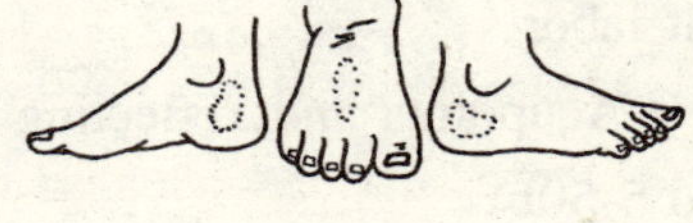

Fig. 5-49b

Manipulation:

1) Pressing and kneading kidney and reproduction reflecting areas on the hand; rubbing central part of the palm and pushing palmar interosseous spaces between metacarpal bones; and kneading and pressing the little finger.

2) Digit-pressing stomach, intestine, kidney, reproduction, urinary bladder and urethra holographic areas on the foot; and rubbing Yongquan (KI 1) acupoint on plantar side of the foot.

3) The gentle moxibustion may be applied at the correlated acupoints and areas and the Le'an No. 3 recipe can be used for hand and foot massage. The manipulation should be quickly and nimbly applied, and sudden manipulation should be avoided. Other therapies for this condition should be applied in combina-

tion, and the patient is advised to visit a gynecologist.

50. Abnormal Position of Fetus

The occipital presentation is the normal fetal position, and the occipitoanterior position is the most common. Otherwise, the occipitoposterior, breech, horizontal, and arm presentations are all abnormal fetal positions, usually discovered in prenatal examinations. They should be corrected in time to avoid difficult labor.

Acupoints and reflecting areas: As shown in Fig. 5-50a and 5-50b.

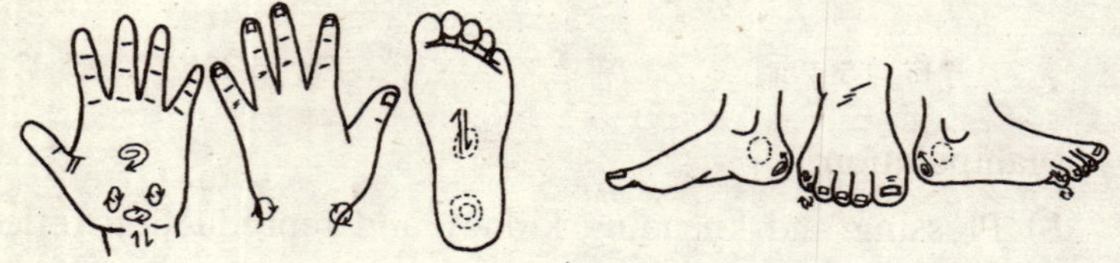

Fig. 5-50a   Fig. 5-50b

Manipulation:

1) Rubbing and twisting Zhiyin (BL 67) acupoint on the foot until a hot sensation is produced, or applying steam therapy and moxibustion.

2) Grinding central part of the palm; and kneading kidney and reproduction holographic areas on the hand; and rubbing proximal part of the palm.

3) Rubbing central part of the sole to produce a hot sensation; digit-pressing kidney, reproduction and uterus holographic

areas on the foot; and grinding of the heel.

4) A hand and foot hot water bath is taken before applying above manipulation, and the hand and foot warmth should be maintained. The manipulation should be gently applied, without any violent and persistent action, and the patient should relax the body and mind and breathe evenly.

51. Reactions After Artificial Abortion

An artificial abortion by uterine curettage and drainage may cause some reactions in pregnant women, including soreness and strain in waist, abdominal distension and pain in lower abdomen of varying severity, and complications such as infection, irregular menstruation and endometriosis.

Acupoints and reflecting areas: As shown in Fig. 5-51a and 5-51b.

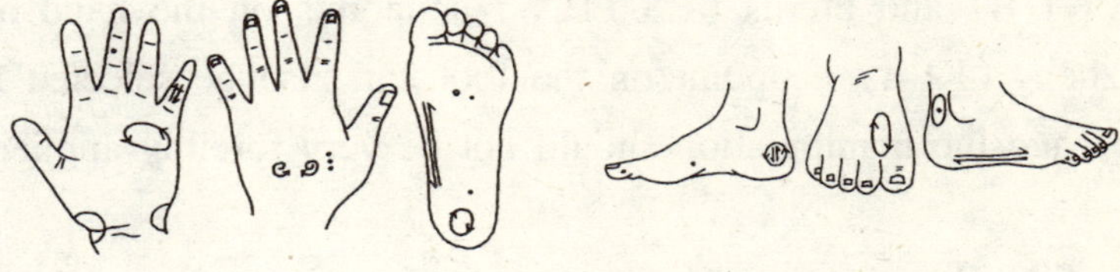

Fig. 5-51a   Fig. 5-51b

Manipulation:

1) Digit-pressing pelvic cavity (EX-PH 22) acupoint on palmar side of the hand, and waist, leg and lower abdomen holographic points on dorsal side of the hand with the proper pressure.

2）Digit-pressing Yongquan（KI 1）, pain-controlling （EX-PF 30）and ear（EX-PF 21）acupoints on plantar side of the foot, and Yinbai（SP 1）, Gongsun（SP 4）, Kunlun（BL 60）and Zhiyin（BL 67）acupoints on dorsal side of the foot with a medium pressure.

3）Gently kneading liver, gallbladder and reproductive gland holographic areas on the hand; and gently grinding waist and leg pain acupoint（EX-DH 3）on dorsal side of the hand.

4）Rubbing medial and lateral borders of the sole until a hot sensation is produced; rubbing and kneading reproductive gland holographic area on medial side of the heel; gently kneading liver and gallbladder holographic areas on dorsal side of the foot; and pressing and kneading pelvic cavity holographic area on lateral malleolus.

5）The Le'an No.1 recipe can be used for foot bath. Shaofu（HT 8）and uterus（EX-PH 5）acupoints on the hand and Dazhong（KI 4）acupoint on the foot can also be selected for use, and the manipulation should not be very forcibly applied.

52. Postpartum Care

Immediately after childbirth, the mother may develop dizziness, blurred vision, cold sweats, irritability, chest distress, shortness of breath; or constipation over several days; or difficult urination and strain of lower abdomen.

According to the traditional Chinese medicine, in about one month after childbirth, the mother usually suffers from a marked deficiency of qi, blood and Jinye (body fluid) and apparent impairment of body resistance. The new mothers are therefore susceptible to attacks of various pathogens, and the resultant diseases may linger over a long time to form a stubborn sickness. This is why postpartum care is particularly emphasized among Chinese people.

Acupoints and reflecting areas: As shown in Fig. 5-52a and 5-52b.

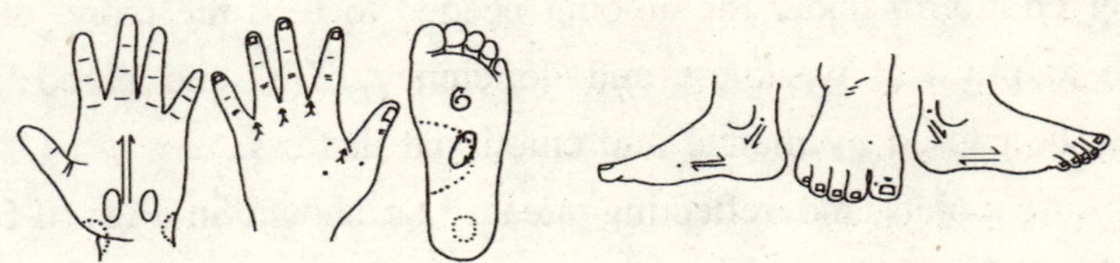

Fig. 5-52a   Fig. 5-52b

1) Digit-pressing brain (EX-DH 14) acupoint, head holographic point and Hegu (LI 4) acupoint on dorsal side of the hand and reproductive gland holographic area on the hand.

2) Digit-pressing kidney, ear, stomach and reproduction holographic areas on the foot; persistently digit-pressing Taixi (KI 3), Gongsun (SP 4), Dadun (LR 1), Taichong (LR 3) and Kunlun (BL 60) acupoints on dorsal side of the foot.

3) Pressing and kneading kidney and urinary bladder holographic areas on the hand; deeply pushing from proximal part of the palm to the middle finger; and heavily pinching web borders of dorsum of the hand.

4) Grinding central part of the sole and pressing and

kneading kidney holographic area on plantar side of the foot;
pushing medial and lateral malleoli; and gently rubbing medial
and lateral borders of the instep.

5) The Le'an No. 1 recipe can be used for foot bath. The
manipulation should be heavily applied for acute symptoms.

53. Hypogalactia

Hypogalactia is the reduction of milk excretion in women
after childbirth under the amount needed to feed the baby. It is
due to physical weakness and deficiency of qi and blood; or
may be caused by mental and emotional distress.

Acupoints and reflecting areas: As shown in Fig. 5-53a
and 5-53b.

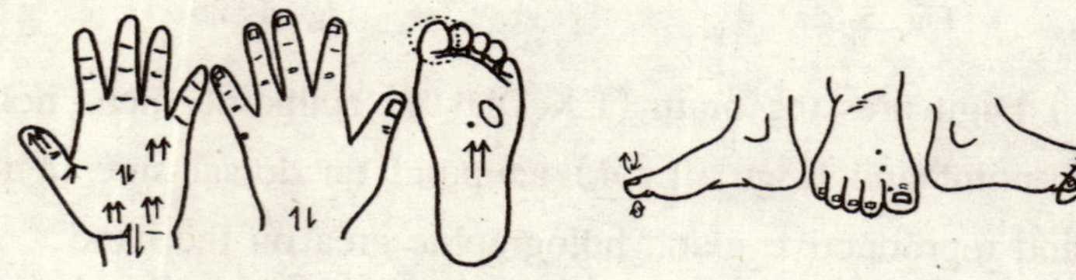

Fig. 5-53a   Fig. 5-53b

Manipulation:

1) Digit-pressing, kneading, twisting and rubbing Shaoze
(SI 1) and Qian'gu (SI 2) on dorsal side of the hand or applying moxibustion and team therapy to them.

2) Digit-pressing Yongquan (KI 1) acupoint on plantar
side of the foot and Taichong (LR 3), Dadun (LR 1) and
Xingjian (LR 2) acupoints on dorsal side of the foot.

3) Pushing and rubbing head, kidney and liver reflecting areas on the hand; and rubbing central and proximal section of the palm.

4) Pushing and pressing kidney, liver and head holographic areas on the foot; twisting and kneading all toes and web borders; and rubbing central part of the sole.

5) The Le'an No. 1 recipe can be used for foot bath. The manipulation should be continuously and properly applied and other acupoints and reflecting areas for other symptoms can also be selected for use.

54. Prolapse of Uterus

In patients with prolapse of uterus, the uterus may descend from its normal position to a level below ischial spine, with some bulge of the anterior and posterior vaginal walls due to loose connective tissue in the pelvic cavity caused by multiple labor or overstraining during childbirth.

Acupoints and reflecting areas: As shown in Fig. 5-54a and 5-54b.

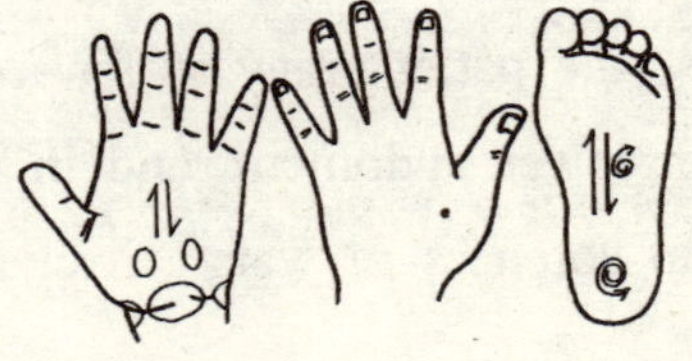

Fig. 5-54a

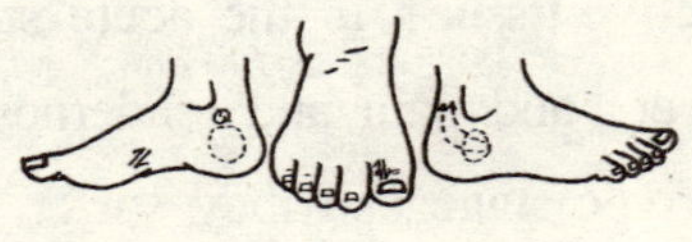

Fig. 5-54b

Manipulation:

1) Rubbing and kneading Dadun (LR 1), Shuiquan (KI 5) and Gongsun (SP 4) acupoints on dorsal side of the foot or applying moxibustion and steam therapy to them; and digit-pressing and kneading lower abdomen holographic point on dorsal side of the hand.

2) Pressing and grinding kidney, uterus and reproduction reflecting areas on the hand and foot; and rubbing and pushing central part of the palm and sole.

3) The Le'an No. 1 and No. 4 recipes can be used for hand and foot bath before above manipulation. The manipulation should be deeply and forcibly applied to improve blood circulation and enhance the repair of connective tissue in the pelvic cavity to correct the prolapsed uterus.

55. Pelvic Inflammation

This is the general term for a condition which includes inflammation of the female reproductive organs in the pelvic—cavity uterus, oviduct and ovary—and their surrounding connective tissue. In the acute stage, the patient may suffer from fever, and pain and tenderness in lower abdomen; and in the chronic stage she may suffer from soreness in waist, irregular menstruation, and infertility.

Acupoints and reflecting areas: As shown in Fig. 5-55a and 5-55b.

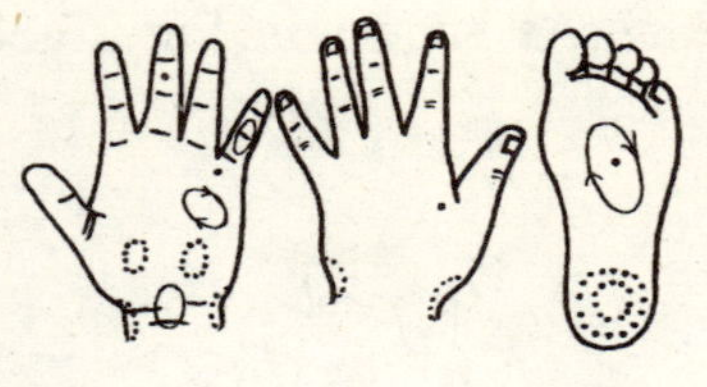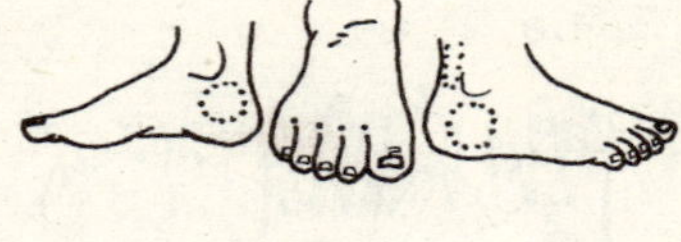

Fig. 5-55a
Fig. 5-55b

Manipulation:

1) Pinching and digit-pressing pelvic cavity (EX-PH 22) and uterus (EX-PH 5) acupoints on palmar side of the hand and lower abdomen holographic point on dorsal side of the hand.

2) Digit-pressing and kneading Yongquan (KI 1) acupoint on plantar side of the foot and Bafeng (EX-DF 3) acupoint on dorsal side of the foot.

3) Pressing and kneading reproduction, ovary, oviduct, uterus, liver and kidney reflecting areas on the hand and foot.

4) The Le'an No. 2 recipe is used for foot bath. The deep and forcible manipulation should be applied for acute inflammation, and medium manipulation for chronic inflammation.

56. Hysteromyoma

Hysteromyoma is a benign tumor composed of muscle and fibrous tissue in the muscular wall of the uterus, most common in women 30-50 years of age. They may suffer from profuse menstrual discharge, irregular uterine bleeding, infertility, abortion with pain, distension, and abdominal mass.

Acupoints and reflecting areas: As shown in Fig. 5-56a and 5-56b.

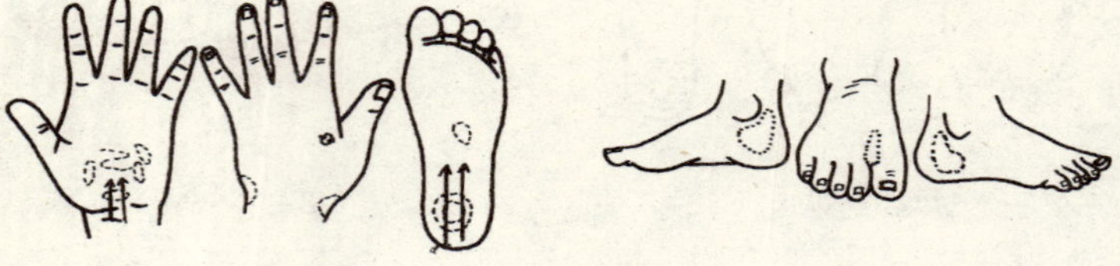

Fig. 5-56a   Fig. 5-56b

Manipulation:

1) Digit-pressing lower abdomen holographic point on the hand and foot.

2) Digit-pressing and kneading kidney, reproduction, intestine and spleen holographic areas on the hand; and pushing proximal section of the palm.

3) Digit-pressing kidney, reproduction and uterus holographic areas on the foot; and pushing plantar side and heel of the foot.

4) The Le'an No. 1 recipe may be used for an extended foot bath. The manipulation should be deeply and forcibly applied and the patients should relax the mind and abdomen. Usually they should practice stomach and breathing exercises.

57. Pruritus Vulva

This is a disease related to the disorder of leukorrhea with symptoms including itching and pain of external genitalia and vagina, sometimes radiated to the anal region and medial sides of the thighs. The patient may also suffer from restlessness at any time, profuse discharge of leukorrhea, irritability, bitter taste in mouth, dizziness, and vertigo.

Acupoints and reflecting areas: As shown in Fig. 5-57a and 5-57b.

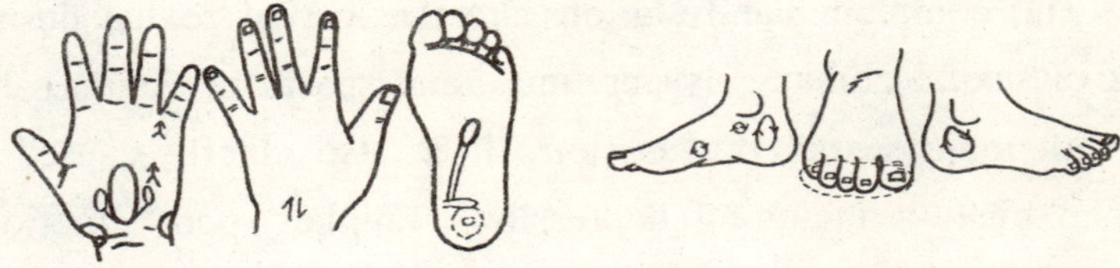

Fig. 5-57a   Fig. 5-57b

Manipulation:

1) Digit-pressing and pinching uterus (EX-PH 5) and Shaofu (HT 8) acupoints on palmar side of the hand.

2) Digit-pressing and kneading Zhaohai (KI 6) and Gongsun (SP 4) acupoints on the foot.

3) Pressing and kneading stomach, intestine, kidney, urinary bladder and reproduction reflecting areas on the hand; and rubbing proximal of the palm.

4) Pressing and kneading reproduction, kidney, urinary bladder and urethra reflecting areas on the foot.

5) The Le'an No. 3 recipe can be used for foot bath. Other acupoints and reflecting areas may be selected according to the symptoms, such as the acupoints and reflecting areas related to the head. For acute and severe itching, the manipulation should be forcibly and deeply applied; but ordinarily it may be

moderately applied. The patient should also take care of their perineal hygiene, for example frequently washing perineal region and changing underwear.

58. Sexual Dysfunction in Women

The common manifestations are the loss of sexual desire, lack of sexual climax, dyspareunia, and spasm of vagina. Just as with male sexual dysfunction, it is also chiefly caused by mental distress including depression, fatigue, poor emotional rapport between couples, unpleasant sexual intercourse, and poor preparation for sexual coition.

Acupoints and reflecting areas: As shown in Fig. 5-58a and 5-58b.

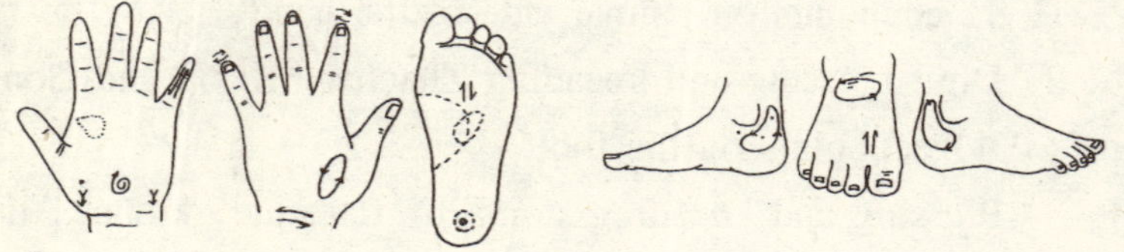

Fig. 5-58a   Fig. 5-58b

1) Digit-pressing endocrine acupoint (EX-PH 3) and liver holographic area, and pincing reproductive gland holographic area on the hand.

2) Digit-pressing Taixi (KI 3), Zhaohai (KI 6) and Shuiquan (KI 5) acupoints on dorsal side of the foot; and heavily digit-pressing kidney, ear, stomach, eye and reproduction holographic areas on plantar side of the foot.

3) Grinding kidney holographic area on palmar side of the hand; pressing and kneading nerve and blood pressure holographic areas on dorsal side of the hand; twisting the index and little fingers; and rubbing palmar side of the little finger and dorsal side of the wrist until producing a hot sensation.

4) Pressing and kneading medial and lateral sides of the ankle joint; rubbing central part of the sole, and pushing liver and gallbladder holographic areas on dorsal side of the foot.

5) The Le'an No. 4 recipe or hot water may be used for hand and foot bath every night before going to bed.

59. Appendicitis

This is a common abdominal surgical disease. At the early stage the patient may suffer from persistent pain in the upper or middle abdomen around the umbilicus with periodic exacerbation. A few hours, or 24 hours later the pain may migrate and localize in the lower right abdomen accompanied by nausea, vomiting, and diarrhea or constipation.

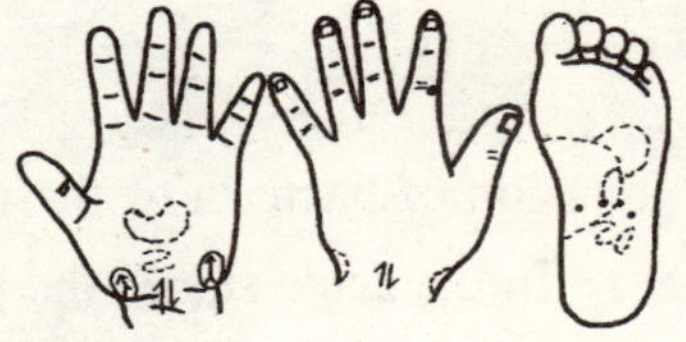

Fig. 5-59a

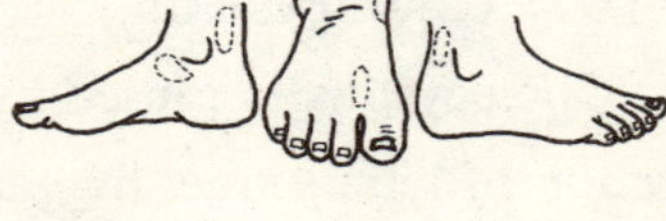

Fig. 5-59b

Acupoints and reflecting areas: As shown in Fig. 5-59a and 5-59b.

Manipulation:

1) Pinching and digit-pressing frontal headache acupoint (EX-DH 6a) on dorsal side of the hand.

2) Digit-pressing and kneading colon (EX-PF 22), small intestine (EX-PF 24), stomach (EX-PF 23) and No. 5 (EX-PF 8) acupoints on plantar side of the foot.

3) Digit-pressing and kneading stomach and intestine holographic areas on the hand; pinching and pressing proximal part of the thenar and hypothenar prominences; and rubbing proximal part of the palm.

4) Digit-pressing and kneading stomach, intestine, appendix, liver and kidney holographic areas on the foot.

5) The Le'an No. 2 and No. 3 recipes can be used for foot bath before applying above manipulation. In the acute stage, the manipulation should be deeply and heavily applied together with other therapies; and in the chronic stage, the medium manipulation may be constantly applied to the related acupoints and reflecting areas.

60. Cholecystitis

Cholecystitis is caused by an invasion of bacteria or the obstruction of biliary tract by gallstones. In the acute stage, the patient may suffer from paroxysmal colic pain of right upper abdomen after a heavy meal, accompanied by apparent local tenderness, spasms of abdominal muscles, vomiting, and fever; and in the chronic stage, they may suffer from dull pain and indigestion.

Acupoints and reflecting areas: As shown in Fig. 5-60a and 5-60b.

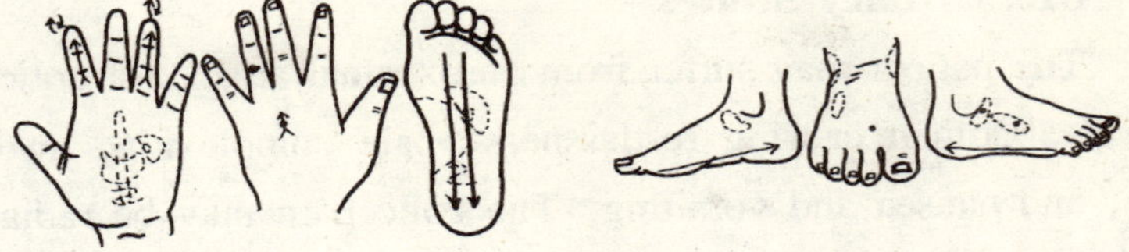

Fig. 5-60a   Fig. 5-60b

Manipulation:

1) Digit-pressing and kneading temporal headache acupoint (EX-PH 6c) on the hand; and in acute stage pinching and digit-pressing Kongji (EX-DH 35) acupoint on dorsal side of the hand.

2) Heavily and persistently digit-pressing and kneading Linqi (GB 41) and Qiuxu (GB 40) acupoints on the foot; and acupoints and reflecting areas for relaxation also can be added for use.

3) Digit-pressing and pushing liver, gallbladder, digestive tract, stomach and intestine reflecting areas on the hand; and twisting and pinching the index and little fingers.

4) Heavily digit-pressing liver, gallbladder, stomach and intestine reflecting areas on the foot; and heavily pushing over the sole from distal end of the foot to the heel.

5) The Le'an No. 2 or No. 3 recipes may be used for foot bath during the chronic stage. In the acute stage, a correct diagnosis should be quickly made for application of heavy manip-

ulation; in chronic cases, the medium manipulation is applied.

61. Urinary Stones

The patient may suffer from paroxysmal attacks of colic in lower abdomen causing restlessness, pale complexion, sweating, and nausea and vomiting. The colic pain may be radiated along the direction of ureter to medial side of thigh and external genitalia, and the stone obstruction in urinary tract may cause retention of urine.

Acupoints and reflecting areas: As shown in Fig. 5-61a and 5-61b.

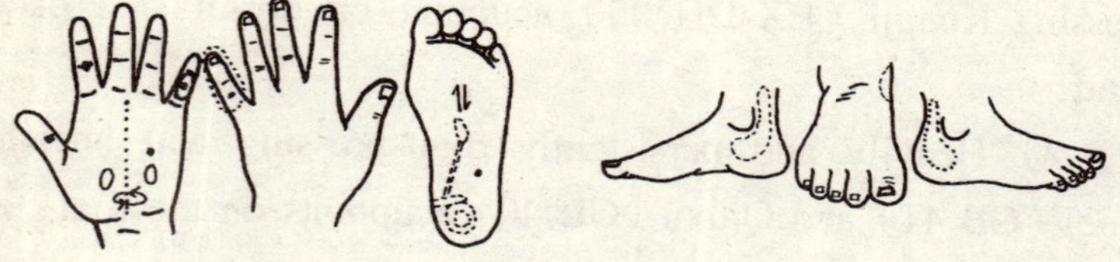

Fig. 5-61a   Fig. 5-61b

Manipulation:

1) Pinching and digit-pressing urethra (EX-PH 15) and Mingmen (EX-PH 20) and Shaofu (HT 8) acupoints on palmar side of the hand.

2) Heavily digit-pressing ear acupoint (EX-PF 21) on plantar side of the foot.

3) Pressing and kneading kidney and urinary bladder reflecting areas on the hand; and pinching and digit-pressing midline of the palm from proximal to distal end.

4) Heavily digit-pressing kidney, ureter, urinary bladder and genital organ reflecting areas on the foot; and rubbing central part of the foot.

5) The Le'an No. 1 recipe can be used the foot bath. For acute attacks, the heavy and deep manipulation should be applied; and during remission, the medium manipulation should be applied. According to the clinical condition, other acupoints and reflecting areas may be added for use, such as the acupoints and reflecting areas for stomach and for retention of urine.

62. Acute Mastitis

This is an infection of the breast occurring after an invasion of bacteria into the mammary gland and ducts producing redness, swelling, hotness, pain and a palpable mass in the breast, swollen lymph nodes in the ipsilateral axillary pit, and pain and general malaise.

Acupoints and reflecting areas: As shown in Fig. 5-62a and 5-62b.

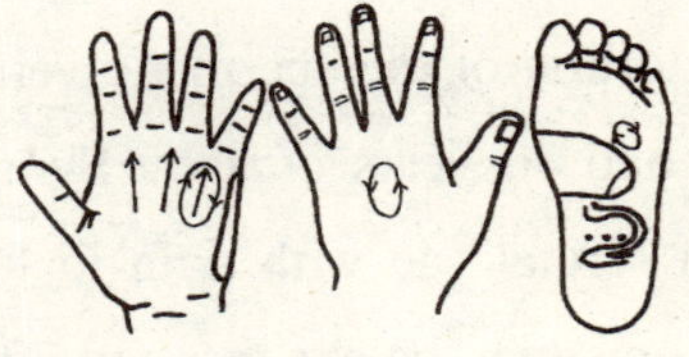

Fig. 5-62a

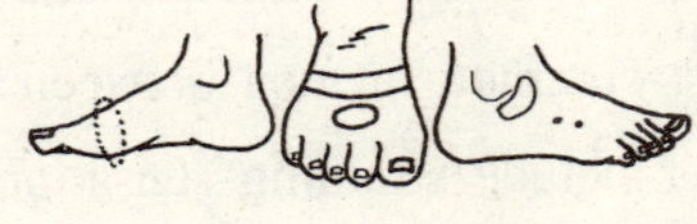

Fig. 5-62b

Manipulation:

1) Heavily digit-pressing 3 Ludi (EX-PF 35) and

Yongquan (KI 1) acupoints on plantar side of the foot.

2) Pressing and kneading Diwuhui (GB 42) and Zulinqi (GB 41) acupoints on dorsal side of the foot; moxibustion or steam therapy may also be applied to them.

3) Pressing and kneading chest, liver, mammary gland and related lymphatic reflecting areas on the hand; and pushing interosseous spaces on dorsal side of the hand.

4) Pressing and kneading chest, liver, mammary gland, kidney, stomach and intestine reflecting areas on the foot; and rubbing midline of the sole.

5) The Le'an No. 2 recipe can be used for a longer hand and foot bath. The manipulation should be deeply and heavily applied, especially to the sensitive spots or sensitive holographic points on the hand and foot. The proper stimulation may be applied during remission to improve the therapeutic effect.

63. Varicocele

This is the elongation and distortion of the spermatic vein, most common in men between 20 and 30 years of age. Symptoms include straining sensation in scrotal sac with pain in left testis and local mass. These symptoms may be exaggerated after standing or walking for a long time.

Acupoints and reflecting areas: As shown in Fig. 5-63a and 5-63b.

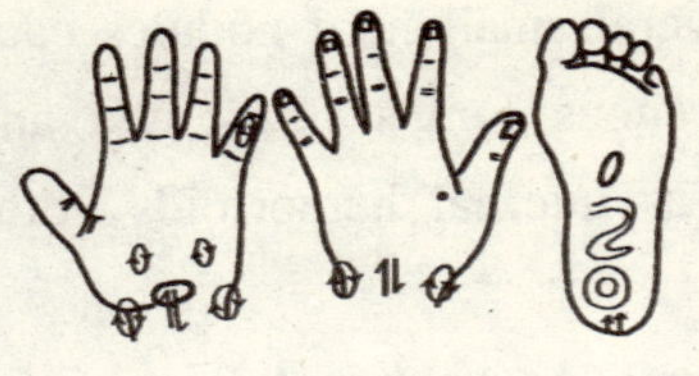
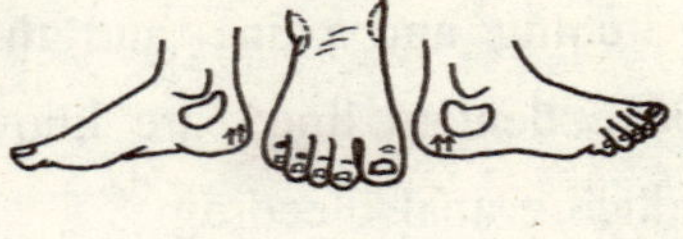

Fig. 5-63a   Fig. 5-63b

Manipulation:

1) Pressing and kneading reproduction, testis and kidney holographic areas on the hand; and rubbing dorsal side of the wrist.

2) Pressing and kneading reproduction, testis, kidney and intestine holographic areas on the foot; and pushing the heel.

3) Digit-pressing sensitive holographic points and areas for diagnosis.

4) The Le'an No. 3 recipe can be used for hand and foot bath. The correspondent acupoints and reflecting areas can also be selected for use in treating this disease.

The hand and foot massage can produce a good therapeutic effect by relieving the discomfort and improving the local blood circulation.

64. Hemorrhoids

Hemorrhoids are venous lumps beneath the mucosa of the distal end of rectum and the skin of anal canal. The venous lumps on the anus (below dentate line) are called external hem-

orroids, which may be one or several small hard nodules causing itching and pain; and the venous lumps inside the anus
(above dentate line) are known as internal hemorroids, often
producing anal bleeding.

Acupoints and reflecting areas: As shown in Fig. 5-64a
and 5-64b.

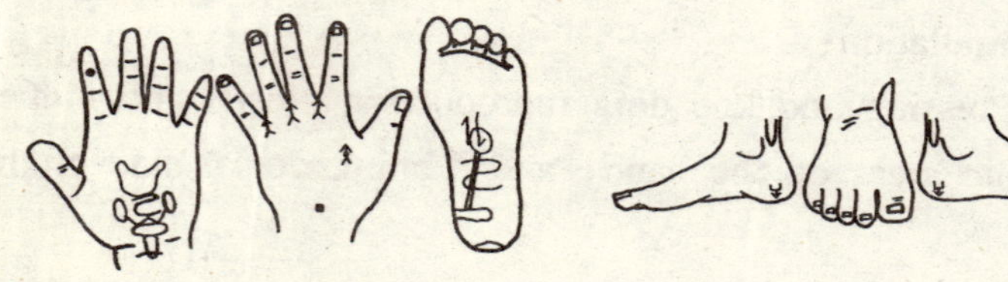

Fig. 5-64a   Fig. 5-64b

Manipulation:

1) Digit-pressing and pinching colon (EX-PH 14) and Yiwofeng (EX-DH 19) acupoints and lower abdomen holographic
point on the hand.

2) Digit-pressing Sugu (BL 65) acupoint on the foot.

3) Pressing and kneading intestine, stomach, anus, kidney
and urinary bladder holographic areas on the hand; and pinching
all web borders.

4) Pressing and kneading anus, intestine, urinary bladder
and kidney reflecting areas on the foot; rubbing central part of
the foot; and stepping on sole.

5) The Le'an No. 1 and No. 3 recipes can be used for

hand and foot bath. The manipulation may be continuously applied to the patient who assumes a prone posture.

65. Cervical Spondylotic Syndrome

The mixed type of this syndrome is most common. The patient may suffer dizziness, headache, numbness and weakness of fingers, and pain in neck and nape radiated to shoulder and one or both arms. Severe cases may develop syncope and paralysis.

Acupoints and reflecting areas: As shown in Fig. 5-65a and 5-65b.

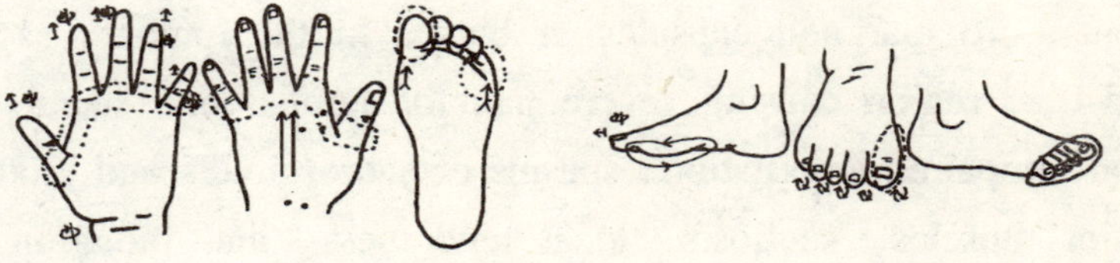

Fig. 5-65a   Fig. 5-65b

Manipulation:

1) Digit-pressing and kneading hypertensing (EX-DH 13), stiff neck (EX-DH 11) and Yangchi (TE 4) acupoints on dorsal side of hand; pulling, rotating, twisting and pinching all fingers and wrist; and pinching nail roots.

2) Pressing and kneading head, shoulder and neck holographic points and areas on the hand; and pushing and pressing

dorsal and bilateral sides of the 3rd metacarpal bone.

3) Heavily digit-pressing shoulder, neck and head reflecting areas on the foot; and twisting, kneading, rotating and pulling all toes, especially the metatarsophalangeal joints of the big and little toes.

4) The Le'an No. 1 and No. 3 recipes can be used for hand and foot bath. The manipulation should be deeply applied and greater manipulation is applied to the affected side. During treatment, the patient should actively rotate his head and neck.

66. Acute Lumbar Sprain

This is an acute soft tissue sprain including muscles, ligaments, articular and capsules or bursae in the lumbar, sacral and iliac region causing severe pain of lumbar and sacral region, impaired ambulation, spasms of sacrospinalis and gluteus major muscles, scoliosis, local tenderness, and radiation of pain to buttocks.

Acupoints and reflecting areas: As shown in Fig. 5-66a and 5-66b.

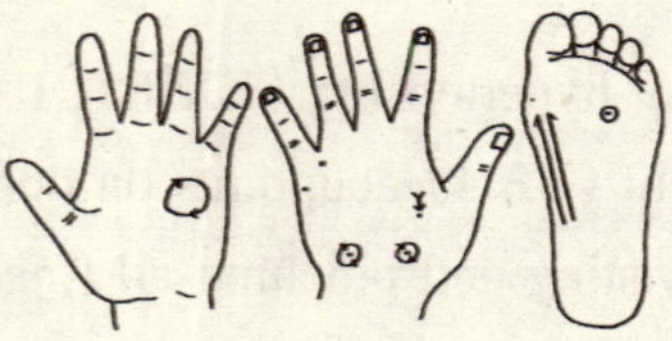

Fig. 5-66a 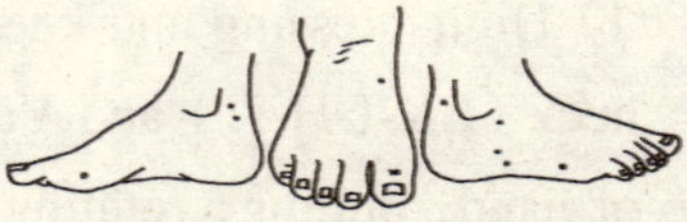   Fig. 5-66b

Manipulation:

1) Kneading waist reflecting area of palmar side of the hand.

2) Heavily pinching waist holographic acupoint beside the metacarpal bone on dorsal side of the hand; digit-pressing and kneading waist and leg pain acupoint (EX-D 6), Jinling and Weiling acupoints), scientic neuralgia (EX-LH 9) and Houxi (SI 3) acupoints on dorsal side of the hand. The patient is asked to move his waist during treatment.

3) Digit-pressing pain-controlling acupoint (EX-PF 30) on plantar side of the foot with deep pressure for a long time; and pushing medial border of the instep to produce a sore and distending sensation.

4) The Le'an No. 4 recipe may be used for foot bath. Digit-pressing and pinching are used as the chief maneuvers for stopping pain and Taixi (KI 3), Dazhong (KI 4), Taibai (SP 3), Kunlun (BL 60), Qiuxu (GB 40), Jinmen (BL 63), Jinggu (BL 64), Sugu (BL 65) and No. 18 acupoint (EX-DF 9) can also be selected for use. The patient should lie flat when resting, and avoid sitting and standing for too long.

67. Furuncles and Furunculosis

The furuncle is a pyogenic infection of a single hair follicle and its appendix. The skin lesion is a small red, swollen, hard and painful nodule. Furunculosis is the simultaneous or repeated appearance of multiple furuncles on certain parts of the body, usually occurring in infants or the malnourished.

acupoints and reflecting areas: As shown in Fig. 5-67a
and 5-67b.

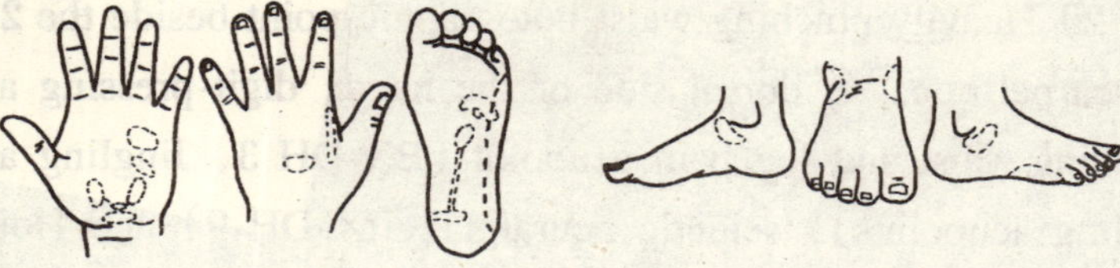

Fig. 5-67a   Fig. 5-67b

Manipulation:

1) Digit-pressing sensitive spots or holographic points on the hand and foot.

2) Digit-pressing spleen, kidney, reproduction and liver holographic areas on the hand.

3) Digit-pressing related lymphatic, liver, kidney, ureter and urinary bladder holographic areas on the foot.

4) The Le'an No. 2 recipe may be used for hand and foot bath or for washing the lesions. The manipulation should be deeply and persistently applied, and other acupoints and reflecting areas for complications may also be selected for use. The hand and foot massage can promote the discharge of toxin and improve the therapeutic effect of drugs.

68. Urticaria

This is an allergic skin disease with the sudden appearance of pink or pale papules of varied size and shape and with severe itching. Urticaria is usually caused by the ingestion of shrimp, crab, drugs or pollen, and it may spontaneously disappear within two weeks.

Acupoints and reflecting areas: As shown in Fig. 5-68a and 5-68b.

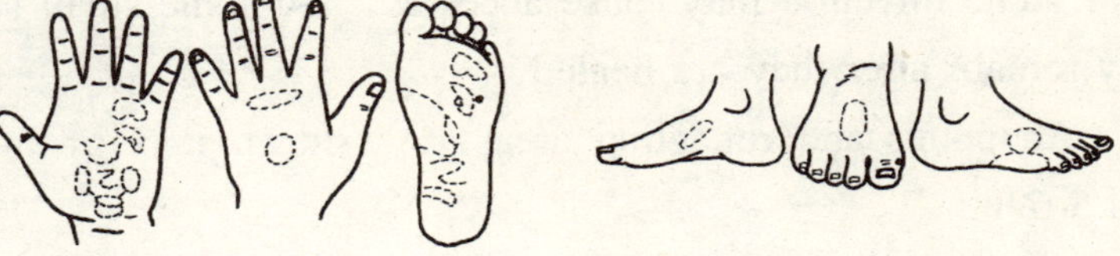

Fig. 5-68a   Fig. 5-68b

Manipulation:

1) Persistently digit-pressing No. 11 acupoint (EX-PF 14) on plantar side of the foot and No. 23 acupoint (EX-DF 14) on dorsal side of the foot.

2) Digit-pressing liver, kidney, urinary bladder, stomach and intestine or lung reflecting areas on the hand.

3) Digit-pressing liver, kidney, urinary bladder, stomach and intestine or lung and respiratory tract reflecting areas on the foot.

4) The Le'an No. 3 recipe can be used for hand and foot bath. The manipulation should be deeply applied. The allergen should discovered in order to select the correct correspondent acupoints and reflecting areas. The hand and foot massage can promote the discharge of allergens and end the allergic reaction.

69. Acne

Acne is most common in both male and female youths. The skin lesions often appear on the forehead, root of nose, regions lateral to eyes and eyebrows, and behind the ears. The typical lesions are small papule with black tips, pinpoint in size. Acne infection may cause abcesses, and some small scars may remain after they are healed.

Acupoints and reflecting areas: As shown in Fig. 5-69a and 5-69b.

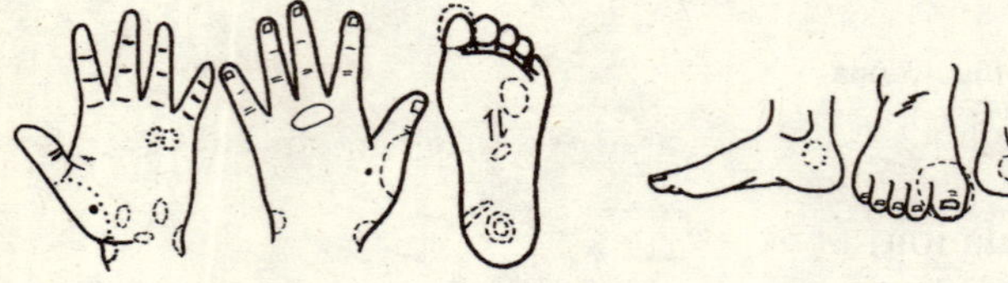

Fig. 5-69a   Fig. 5-69b

Manipulation:

1) Digit-pressing Hegu (LI 4) acupoint and heart, lung, kidney and related reproductive organ areas on the hand; and pinching and digit-pressing endocrine acupoint (EX-PH 3) on palmar side of the hand.

2) Digit-pressing and pinching Qiaoyin (GB 44) acupoint and kneading Yongquan (KI 1) acupoint on the foot; digit-pressing lung, head, reproduction, testis, kidney and urinary bladder reflecting areas on the foot.

3) The Le'an No. 1 and No. 3 recipes may be used for hand and foot bath. The manipulation should be moderately and

persistently applied. The related acupoints and reflecting areas of stomach and circulatory system may also be selected for use. The patient should follow a regular regimen of diet and daily life, and avoid eating spicy food.

70. Oral Aphtha

Oral aphthae are ulcerated white blisters occurring on the cheeks, lips and tongue causing redness, swelling, pain, and low fever. They may fuse together to form a large ulcerative surface producing intolerable pain and difficulty speaking, and eating and drinking.

Acupoints and reflecting areas: As shown in Fig. 5-70a and 5-70b.

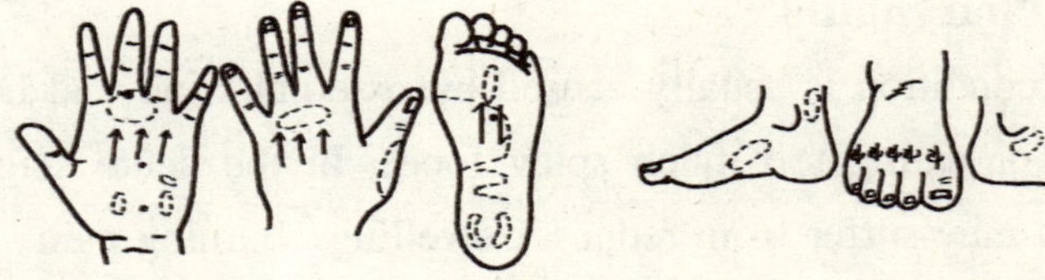

Fig. 5-70a   Fig. 5-70b

Manipulation:

1) Pinching and digit-pressing aphtha (EX-PH 11), Nei-yangchi (EX-PH 28) and Laogong (PC 8) acupoints on palmar side of the hand.

2) Digit-pressing and kneading Yongquan (KI 1) acupoint on plantar side of the foot.

3) Digit-pressing mouth, spleen and kidney reflecting ar-

eas and related positive spots as diagnosed on the hand; and pushing palm and fingers.

4) Heavily rubbing the sole; rotating ankle joint and all toes; and digit-pressing and kneading oral cavity, digestive tract, and stomach and intestine holographic areas on the foot.

5) The Le'an No. 3 recipe can be used for hand and foot bath before applying above manipulation. The manipulation should be persistently applied with force and other necessary acupoints and reflecting areas, such as acupoints and reflecting areas of the endocrinal organs, may also be selected for use. Oral hygiene should be maintained and the diet may need to be adjusted.

71. Pharyngitis

This condition is usually caused by external wind and heat pathogens or eating too much spicy food. In the acute stage, the patient may suffer from redness, swelling, burning pain, an obstructive sensation in throat, difficulty swallowing, and hoarseness. It may develop into the chronic stage if not effectively cured in time.

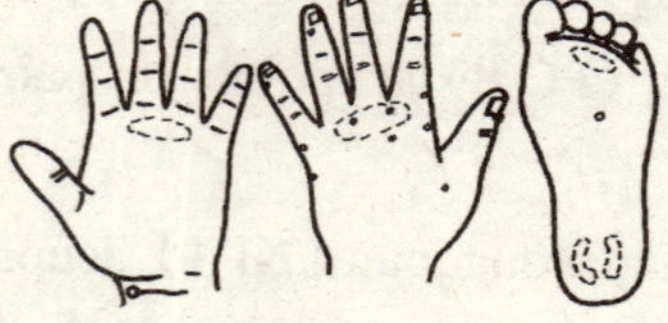

Fig. 5-71a   Fig. 5-71b

Acupoints and reflecting areas: As shown in Fig. 5-71a and 5-71b.

Manipulation:

1) Pinching and pressing Taiyuan (LU 9) acupoint on palmar side of the hand and sore throat (EX-DH 10), Shaoshang (LU 11), Erjian (LI 2), Sanjian (LI 3), Hegu (LI 4), Qian'gu (SI 2), Shaoze (SI 1), Guanchong (TE 1), Zhongzhu (TE 3) and Yemen (TE 2) acupoints on dorsal side of the hand.

2) Digit-pressing Yongquan (KI 1) acupoint on plantar side of the foot and Taixi (KI 3) and Zhaohai (KI 6) acupoints on dorsal side of the foot.

3) Digit-pressing and kneading pharynx and oral cavity reflecting areas on the hand.

4) Digit-pressing pharynx and oral cavity reflecting areas on the foot.

5) The Le'an No. 2 recipe can be used for hand and foot bath before applying above manipulation. The manipulation should be heavily applied in the acute stage; and persistently and forcibly applied in the chronic stage.

72. Toothache

Toothache is a common symptom of various diseases of the oral cavity such as pulpitis, peridentitis, pericoronitis, alveolar abscess, and trigeminal neuralgia.

Acupoints and reflecting areas: As shown in Fig. 5-72a and 5-72b.

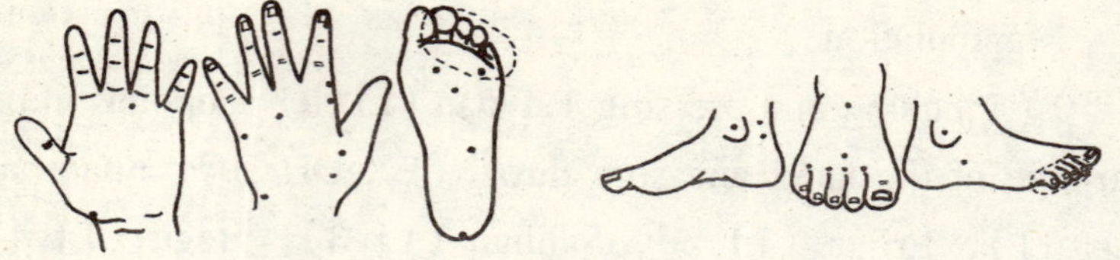

Fig. 5-72a   Fig. 5-72b

Manipulation:

1) Pinching and digit-pressing common cold (EX-PH 25) and toothache (EX-PH 7) acupoints on palmar side of the hand and Shangyang (LI 1), Hegu (LI 4), Erjian (LI 2), Sanjian (LI 3), Yangxi (LI 5), Houxi (SI 3), Shanghegu (EX-DH 9) and Tongling (EX-DH 36) acupoints on dorsal side of the hand.

2) Pinching and digit-pressing No. 12 (EX-PF 15), No. 13 (EX-PF 16), small intestine (EX-PF 24), kidney (EX-PF 33) and Nuxi (EX-PF 3) acupoints on plantar side of the foot and Bafeng (EX-DF 3), Neiting (ST 44), Taixi (KI 3), tip of medial malleolus (EX-DF 1), tip of lateral malleolus (EX-DF 2), Dazhong (KI 4), Jinmen (BL 63) and Chongyang (ST 42) acupoints on dorsal side of the foot.

3) Kneading, digit-pressing, pinching and pressing tooth and oral cavity holographic areas on the foot; and rotating and twisting all toes.

4) The Le'an No. 2 recipe can be used for foot bath before

treatment. The manipulation should be deeply and forcibly applied during an attack of toothache and moderately applied after the toothache subsides. Good oral hygiene should be maintained.

73. Rhinitis

Rhinitis is caused by the invasion of bacteria into the nasal mucosa after repeated bouts of the common cold. Ordinarily, the patient has nasal obstruction in cold weather, heavy breathing and purulent nasal discharge; and during an attack of rhinitis they may suffer from nasal itching, clear nasal discharge, and dizziness and headache in severe cases.

Acupoints and reflecting areas: As shown in Fig. 5-73a and 5-73b.

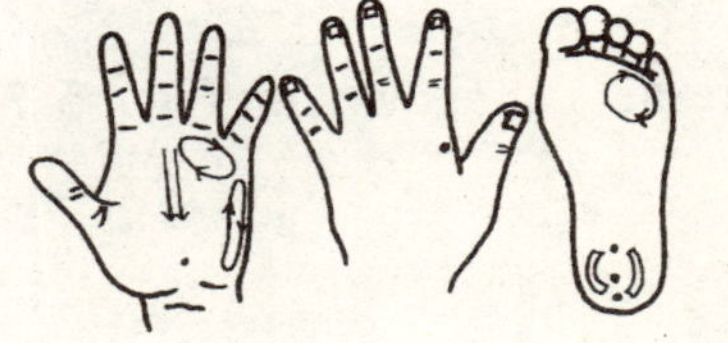

Fig. 5-73a

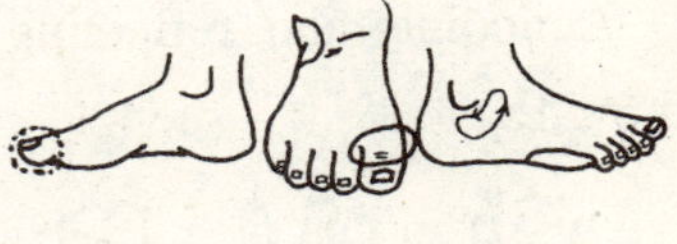

Fig. 5-73b

Manipulation:

1) Pinching and digit-pressing stomach and intestine pain acupoint (EX-PH 8) on palmar side of the hand and head holographic point on dorsal side of the hand.

2) Pinching and digit-pressing No. 1 (EX-PF 4) and regeneration (EX-PF 18) acupoints on dorsal side of the foot.

3) Digit-pressing and kneading nose, pharynx, lung and related lymphatic holographic areas on the hand; pushing middle finger and along midline of the palm.

4) Digit-pressing and kneading nose, pharynx and related lymphatic holographic areas on the foot.

5) The Le'an No. 2 recipe can be used for hand and foot bath. The pressure may be gradually increased to a deep and forceful manipulation.

74. Otitis Media

The onset of otitis media is usually very sudden and the patient may suffer from an obstructive sensation in the ear, hearing impairment, tinnitus, deafness, occasional discharge of pus from ear, fever, thirst, dry mouth, dark urine, and constipation.

Acupoints and reflecting areas: As shown in Fig. 5-74a and 5-74b.

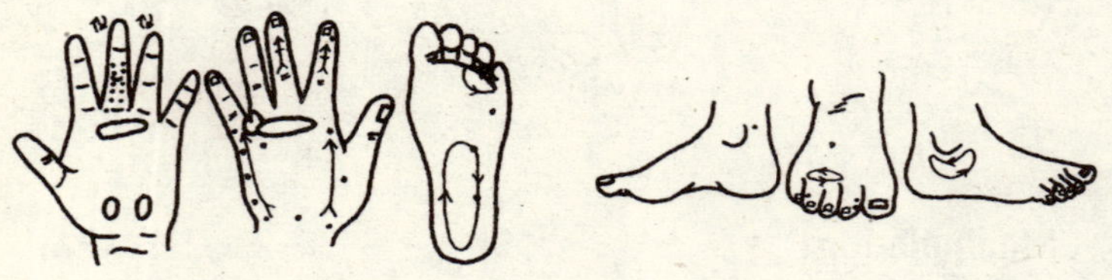

Fig. 5-74a   Fig. 5-74b

Manipulation:

1) Pinching and kneading Shangyang (LI 1), Hegu (LI

4), Yangxi (LI 5), Qian'gu (SI 2), Houxi (SI 3), Shanghouxi (EX-DH 29), Wan'gu (SI 4), Yanggu (SI 5), Zhongzhu (TE 3), Yangchi (TE 4) and head holographic point on
dorsal side of the hand.

2) Pinching and kneading triple energizer (EX-PF 27) and
gallbladder (EX-PF 34) acupoints on plantar side of the foot
and Taixi (KI 3), Zuqiaoyin (GB 44), No. 19 (EX-DF 10),
No. 24 (EX-DF 15) and Qingtou 1 (EX-DF 26) acupoints on
dorsal side of the foot; and digit-pressing ear acupoint (EX-PF
21) on plantar side of the foot for patients with severe pain.

3) Digit-pressing pharynx, ear, lung, intestine and stomach reflecting areas on the hand; twisting and pinching the middle and ring fingers.

4) Digit-pressing and kneading ear, pharynx, kidney and
urinary bladder holographic areas on the foot; and pinching and
kneading 3rd and 4th toes and their metatarsophalangeal joints.

5) The Le'an No. 2 recipe can be used for hand and foot
bath before treatment. The manipulation should be forcefully
and evenly applied and the stronger stimulation may be applied
to the sensitive spots.

75. Myopia

Myopia is a congenital eye condition with abnormal eye-
balls, or acquired after birth due to poor hygiene. Vision may
be improved if proper eyes care or treatment of this condition is
begun in early childhood.

Acupoints and reflecting areas: As shown in Fig. 5-75a and 5-75b.

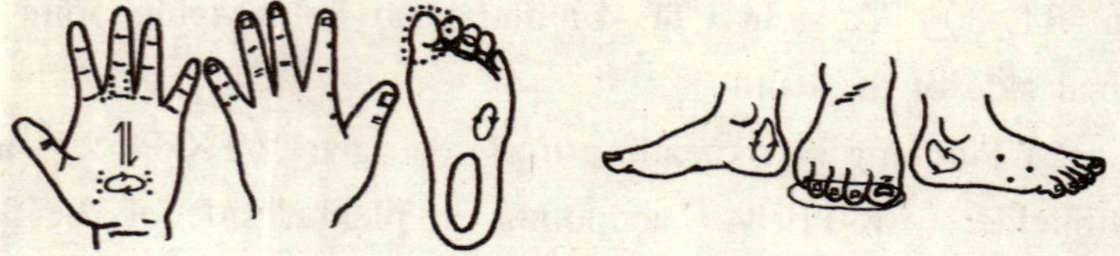

Fig. 5-75a   Fig. 5-75b

Manipulation:

1) Digit-pressing and pinching Erjian (LI 2), Dagukong (EX-DH 20), Xiaogukong (EX-DH 21) and Erming (EX-DH 42) acupoints on dorsal side of the hand; and kneading 3 Jianli acupoints (EX-PH 31) on palmar side of the hand and head holographic point on dorsal side of the hand.

2) Digit-pressing and kneading Linqi (GB 41), Xiaxi (GB 43), Shuiquan (KI 5) and Sugu (BL 65) on dorsal side of the foot.

3) Digit-pressing and kneading eye and kidney reflecting areas on the hand; and rubbing midline of the palm.

4) Digit-pressing head, eye, kidney, liver and reproduction reflecting areas on the foot.

5) The Le'an No. 1 recipe or clean water may be used for foot bath. The medium manipulation is applied and the patient, during treatment, should close his eyes, concentrate attention on the eyes, and move them in various directions.

76. Glaucoma

Glaucoma is characterized by an increase of intraocular pressure, and the patient may suffer from headache, slight eye distension, and impaired vision. The severity of the headache may gradually increased accompained by nausea, vomiting, congestion of conjunctiva, opaque cornea, and eventually blindness, if not effectively treated over a long period of time.

Acupoints and reflecting areas: As shown in Fig. 5-76a and 5-76b.

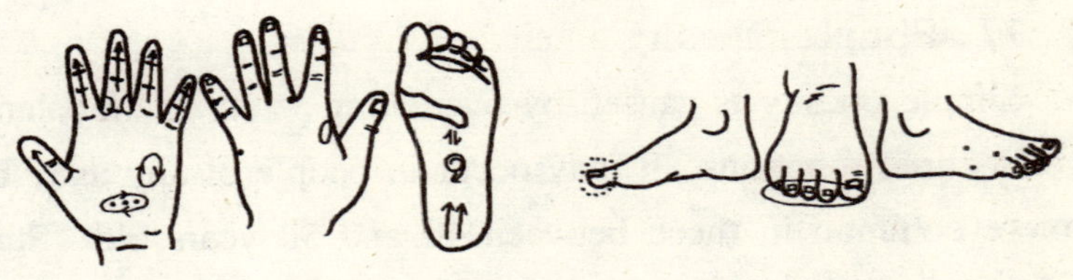

Fig. 5-76a   Fig. 5-76b

Manipulation:

1) Digit-pressing and kneading 3 Jianli acupoints (EX-PH 31) on palmar side of the hand and Erming (EX-DH 42), Dagukong (EX-DH 20), Xiaogukong (EX-DH 21) and antifebrile (EX-DH 43) acupoints, Shangyang (LI 1), Shaoze (SI 1) and Houxi (SI 3) on dorsal side of the hand.

2) Digit-pressing and kneading Linqi (GB 41), Xiaxi (GB 43) and Sugu (BL 65) on dorsal side of the foot.

3) Pushing and grinding eye, liver and kidney holographic

areas on the hand; and pushing palmar, radial and ulnar sides of all fingers.

4) Digit-pressing head, eye, heart and kidney reflecting areas on the foot, ankle joint, heel and sole; and rubbing Yongquan (KI 1) acupoint on plantar side of the foot.

5) The Le'an No. 3 recipe can be used for foot bath before treatment. The manipulation should be moderately and persistently applied and the patient with eyes closed should concentrate attention on the eyes while being treated.

77. Simple Obesity

Simple obesity is caused by overeating, with no imbalance of endocrinal functions. It may occur in people of any age, but is more common in those between 40 and 50 years old. Standard body weight can be calculated as (kg) = [body height (cm) − 100] × 0.9, and simple obesity may be diagnosed if weight is 20% more than the standard weight.

Acupoints and reflecting areas: As shown in Fig. 5-77a and 5-77b.

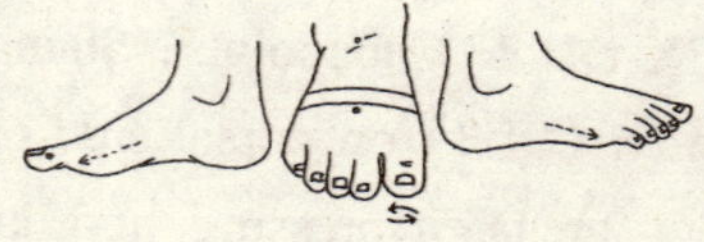

Fig. 5-77a   Fig. 5-77b

Manipulation:

1) Pressing the pads of the thumb and index finger and Hegu (LI 4) acupoint with a moderate pressure for a long time.

2) Heavily pressing Yinbai (SP 1), Jiexi (ST 41) and Xian'gu (ST 43) on dorsal side of the foot.

3) Grinding stomach holographic area on palmar side of the hand; gently kneading thenar prominence; pushing from central to proximal part of the palm and from distal to proximal end of the index finger along its dorsal side; and twisting the thumb.

4) Pressing and kneading plantar side of all toes and diaphragm holographic area on dorsal side of the foot; pushing stomach holographic area on plantar side of the foot; twisting the big toe; digit-pressing and pushing inferior border of medial and lateral metatarsal bones; and stepping on the heel.

5) The Le'an No. 4 recipe may be used for foot bath. The patient should be placed on an adequate diet regimen.

78. Chronic Alcoholism

Chronic alcoholism is the result of excessive consumption of alcoholic drinks over a long time causing damage to the internal organs, especially the liver. The patient may suffer from poor memory, mental confusion, loss of steady movement, poor appetite, tremors, loss of weight, fatigue, and liver palms.

Acupoints and reflecting areas: As shown in Fig. 5-78a and 5-78b.

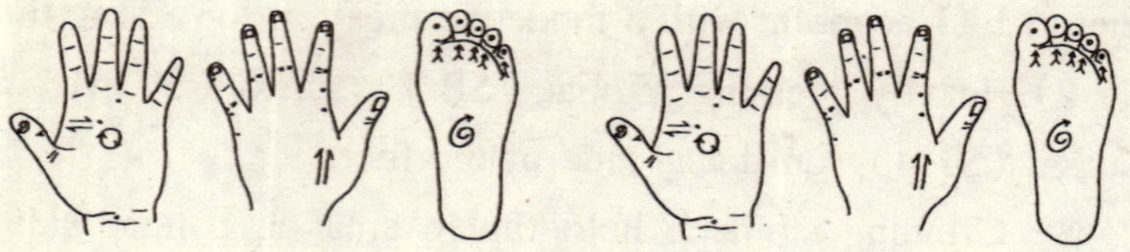

Fig. 5-78a   Fig. 5-78b

Manipulation:

1) Digit-pressing Laogong (PC 8), Daling (PC 7) and spleen (EX-PH 17) acupoints on palmar side of the hand and Shaoze (SI 1), Qian'gu (SI 2), Houxi (SI 3), Shangyang (LI 1), Erjian (LI 2), Sanjian (LI 4) and headache acupoint (EX-DH 6) on dorsal side of the hand with heavy and deep manipulation.

2) Digit-pressing Yinbai (SP 1), Dadu (SP 2), Taibai (SP 3) and Gongsun (SP 4) on dorsal side of the foot; pressing pads of all toes with persistent pressure; and heavily pinching proximal part of all toes.

3) Grinding pad of the thumb; kneading stomach holographic area and rubbing liver holographic area on palmar side of the hand, and pushing nerve and blood pressure holographic areas on dorsal side of the hand.

4) Grinding stomach holographic area on plantar side of the foot; pushing lower border of the first metatarsal bone; pressing and kneading diaphragm, liver and gallbladder holo-

graphic areas on dorsal side of the foot and dorsal side of all toes; rotating ankle joint; and pulling all toes.

5) The Le'an No. 4 recipe may be used for foot bath. The patient should perform hand exercises.

79. Addiction to Tobacco

This is similar to drug addiction. Going without smoking may cause general weakness, poor appetite, mental confusion, and incapacity for the normal activities of daily life. These symptoms are relieved by smoking tobacco. Because of prolonged smoking the patient may also suffer from cough, profuse sputum, poor pulmonary ventilation, heart palpitations, and chest distress.

Acupoints and reflecting areas: As shown in Fig. 5-79a and 5-79b.

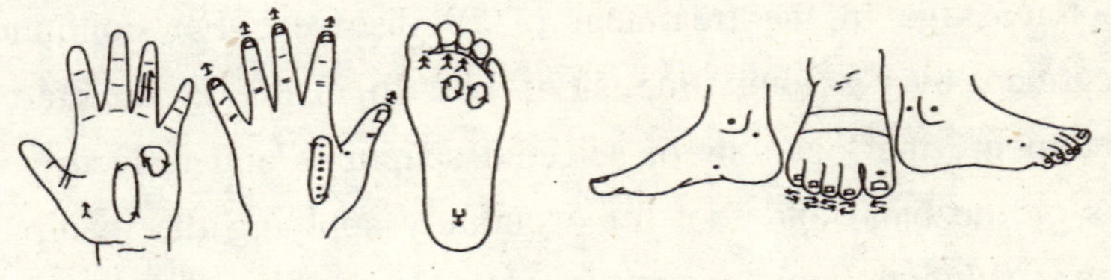

Fig. 5-79a   Fig. 5-79b

Manipulation:

1) Heavily pinching endocrine acupoint (EX-PH 3) on palmar side of the hand and digit-pressing brain acupoint (EX-DH 14) on dorsal side of the hand.

2) Pressing tips of medial malleolus (EX-DF 1) and lateral

malleolus (EX-DF 2) acupoints; digit-pressing Dazhong (KI 4), Ran'gu (KI 2), Kunlun (BL 60), Diwuhui (GB 42), Xia-xi (GB 43) and Zuqiaoyin (GB 44) on the foot; and stepping on the heel.

3) Rubbing the ring finger; pressing and kneading liver, gallbladder, stomach and intestine holographic areas on palmar side of the hand; digit-pressing Hegu (LI 4) acupoint on dorsal side of the hand; and pulling joints of all fingers.

4) Pressing and kneading lung and diaphragm holographic areas on the foot; heavily pinching proximal end of the big, 2nd and 3rd toes; and twisting all toes.

5) The Le'an No. 2 recipe can be used for foot bath. The manipulation at Hegu (LI 4) acupoint on dorsal side of the hand is the most important procedure.

In the foregoing we have considered the use of hand and foot massage in the treatment of 79 diseases. For continuous treatment over a long time, it is best to mark, at the start of treatment, the locations of selected acupoints and reflecting areas on the hand and foot for accurately applying the manipulation. Although some acupoints and reflecting areas appearing in the treatment of a few diseases have not been shown in the figures and diagrams in Chapter 2, their exact locations can be defined from the figures contained in the context of those diseases in this chapter, and by detecting the tender spots in the defined location. The charts prepared by different scholars to show the location of acupoints and reflecting areas for hand and foot massage vary greatly, although they are all praised as the orthodox charts by their authors. However, similar therapeutic effects can be obtained by adopting any one of them because all useful charts were prepared according to the same traditional principle of remote treatment: "To cure diseases in the upper body, apply treatment to the lower body, and vice versa." This principle can also be used regarding the holographic reflecting points and areas. The reflecting area of the middle part of the trunk of the body should be assigned the center of the sole, and the reflecting area of head may be defined either at the distal or the proximal end of the sole. This is why differing acupoints and reflecting areas charts for hand and foot massage can produce similar therapeutic result. The effectiveness of clinical practice is the demonstration of truth. Therefore, the truly orthodox charts will be revealed by successful clinical practice, and the useless charts will be eventually discarded. The hand and foot massage is a concise therapy, and anyone may become proficient at it after continuous learning and scientific practice. The reader may learn much not included in this book from their own clinical practice, and become a health care expert themselves.

CHAPTER 6　HAND AND FOOT MASSAGE FOR COSMETICS AND HEALTH CARE

I. Cosmetics and Health Care

People may first think of plastic surgery and making double-fold eyelids and high nose bridges when they think of cosmetology. Of course, some people find it necessary to improve their appearance. However, for the vast majority of people cosmetology means only maintaining a natural and a good constitution, full of energy and vitality.

As we have said, the hand and foot are closely related to the head. It is common sense that people with normal and proportional hands and feet may correspondently have a health and proportionate body, handsome and charming. So the hand and foot are closely related to cosmetics and health care, and a regular and persistent application of hand and foot massage can improve the looks and maintain the health.

1. Procedures for massage and hand exercise
Procedures for hand massage:

1) Mutually rubbing both hands

The palms of the hands are placed face to face and then rub against each other from low to high speed and again to low speed, repeatedly, until a hot sensation is produced; the fingers of both hands are interlaced and then rub against each other, with the fingers sliding over the web borders from low speed to high speed, and again to low speed, repeatedly; and finally, one palm is used to rub the dorsum of the other hand and wrist and then the hands are switched alternately.

2) Pushing fingers and palm:

The pad or radial corner of distal phalanx of the thumb of one hand is used to rub the fingers of the other hand from radial to ulnar side and from palmar to dorsal side; and then is used to rub the radial border, ulnar border, and proximal of the palm, palmar interosseous spaces, proximal of dorsum of the hand, and dorsal interosseous spaces, sequentially.

3) Twisting and pressing joints:

All joints of the hand and wrist on one side are separately twisted and pressed by the other hand according to the sequence from radial side to ulnar side, and from distal end to proximal end, and then the manipulation is alternately performed on both hands.

4) Pulling and rotating fingers and wrist:

The wrist and all fingers from radial side to ulnar side of one hand are pulled and rotated by the other hand, and then the manipulation is performed alternately on both hands.

5) Pinching and kneading tips of fingers:

The tips and nail roots of all fingers of one hand are pinched and kneaded by the other hand; and the pads of all distal phalanx are kneaded. The manipulation is alternately and repeatedly applied to both hands.

6) Digit-pressing and grinding central part of palm:

The central part of one palm is digit-pressed and grinded by the other hand until a hot sensation is produced, and the manipulation is performed alternately to both palms.

7) Particular adjustment:

The correspondent reflecting areas of the involved organs are particularly pressed and grinded to adjust the dysfunction of these organs.

8) Rubbing palms for adjustment:

The first manipulation is repeated as the closing step in this set of manipulations.

Hand exercise:

1) Expanding fingers and clenching hand:

The fingers are extended and widely separated from each other and then quickly clenched to make a fist. This movement is repeated 200 times.

2) Rolling up nose of an elephant:

The hand is pronated with the palm facing downward and all fingers are extended and expanded, then the little, ring, middle, and index fingers and thumb are flexed in sequence to form a hollow fist while the wrist is half rotated; then the fingers are again extended in the same sequence to resume the starting posture. These movements are repeated 100-200 times with the speed gradually increased. The next finger should start flexing or extending immediately after the prior finger has completely finished its movement. The movement is just like an elephant rolling its nose.

3) Rotating wrist joint to its limit:

The wrist joint rotates either clockwise or counterclockwise with the joint flexed to dorsal, ulnar, ventral and radial sides to the limit, 100-200 times; the hands may be alternately or simultaneously rotated.

In addition, supplemental instruments, like health balls and bracelet may be used for regular hand exercises. The pressing, grinding, hammering, knocking and beating maneuvers may be applied to the palm and dorsum of the hand or the dorsum of the hand may be used to beat the tree. Before these exercises, the hands should be soaked in hot water and dried with a towel. The intensity of exercise should be adequate, and the joints and skin of the hand should be properly protected from injury.

2. Massage procedures and foot exercise

Procedures for foot massage:

1) Rubbing all over the foot:

The feet are placed flat and both hands are used to rub the medial and lateral sides, the instep, the spaces between toes, and finally the sole of the foot, first horizontally and then vertically until a hot sensation is produced.

2) Separately pushing instep and sole of the foot:

Both hands are used to separately push downward from the leg above the medial and lateral malleoli and over the instep until reaching the toes, and then to push downward from the lateral border of the heel over the sole to the toes. The pushing maneuver should be repeatedly applied to the heel.

3) Twisting and pressing joints:

All joints of the foot and ankle are twisted and pressed in a sequence from the big toe to the little toe, and again from distal interphalangeal joints to metatarsophalangeal joints, and then to the ankle joint. A heavier manipulation should be applied to the toes.

4) Pulling and rotating toes and ankle joint:

The pulling and rotating manipulations are applied to the toes following the sequence from the big toe to the little toe and finally to the ankle joint. The rotating manipulation should be applied over the widest range of motion for each joint.

5) Pinching and kneading the tips of toes:

The pinching and kneading maneuvers are applied to the tip, pad and nail root of each toe from the big toe to the little toe. The heavier manipulation should be applied to the big toe.

6) Digit-pressing and grinding central part of sole:

Quickly digit-press and grind central part of the sole to produce a hot sensation.

7) **Particular adjustment**:

The pressing and grinding manipulation is applied to the reflecting areas of involved organs to adjust their functions. Greater adjusting manipulation should be applied to the big toe, the first metatarsophalangeal joint, the region beneath the foot arch, and ankle joint.

8) Rubbing foot for adjustment:

The rubbing foot manipulation is repeated for adjustment as the closing step in this set of manipulations.

Foot exercise:

1) Flexing and extending toes:

All toes are plantarly flexed simultaneously to the limit of movement and then quickly dorsiflexed, also to the limit, in one repitition of exercise, and 100-200 repititions should be performed.

2) Mutually contacting and rubbing toes:

The big and second toes of both feet are kept close together to rub each other 100-200 times, with the range and rubbing frequency gradually increased.

3) Walking on toes or heel:

The practitioner may walk for a while on toes and metatarsophalangeal joints with the heels raised up from the ground; and then walk for a while on heels with the soles raised up from the ground. They may then walk alternately on toes and on heels.

4) Actively rotating ankle joints:

The practitioner may stand on one foot and raise the other foot to rotate the ankle joint clockwise and counterclockwise alternately 100 times, and then this exercise is performed on both ankle joints alternately.

In addition, the pebble container and sand container may be used for foot exercise with bare feet; the pressing, grinding, hammering, knocking and beating maneuvers may be applied all over the foot; and instep, medial and lateral borders of foot may be used to kick a substance. Before the application of manipulation and foot exercise, it is best to soak the feet in hot water and then dry them with a towel. The intensity of exercise should be gentle enough to avoid injuring the joints, ligaments, muscles, and skin.

Self-massage and hand and foot exercise for half an hour every day is very useful for relieving fatigue , restoring vital energy, maintaining body weight, preventing diseases, and slowing the aging process. It may produce a good therapeutic effect in treating obesity, poor memory and sexual dysfunction. In the beginning, doing self-massage and exercise may seems very tedious and strenuous, but it can produce many new and comfortable feelings after persistent practice, if done correctly by following the given requirements.

II. Child Health Care

Health care and medical therapy for children is a special

branch of medicine. Pediatric departments were in use in ancient China, and pediatric massage was separated from massage for adults, much welcomed by the vast Chinese people. The hand and foot massage for the health care of children is introduced as follows:

1. Hand massage for child health care:

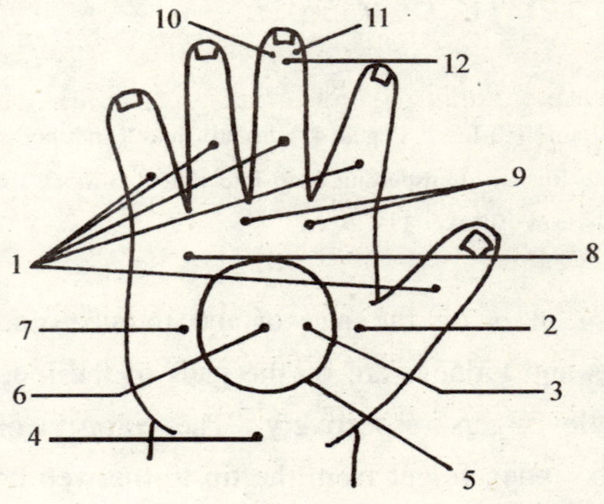

Fig. 6-1

1-Wuzhijie (five interphalangeal joints) 2-Hegu (LI 4) 3-Weiling 4-Yiwofeng 5-Outer Bagua 6-Outer Laogong 7-Jingning 8-Shangmen 9-Ershanmen 10-Right Duanzheng 11-Laolong 12-Left Duanzheng.

The acupoints and areas on the hands of children (Fig . 6 - 1 ,

6-2 and 6-3) are different from those of adults.

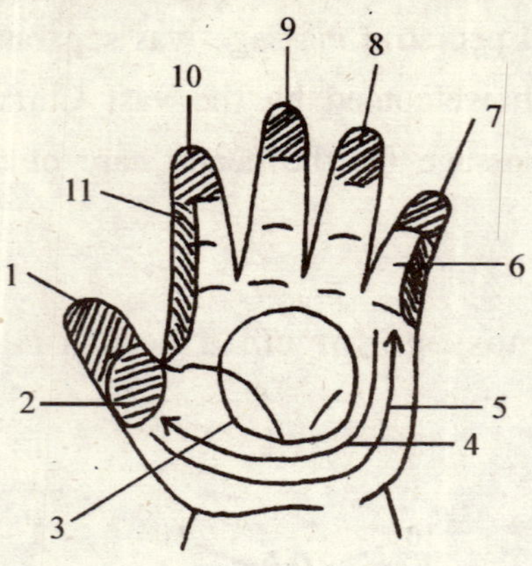

Fig. 6-2

1-Spleen 2-Stomach 3-Inner Bagua 4-Yunshui Rutu (transporting water into earth) 5-Yuntu Rushui (transporting earth into water) 6-Small intestine 7-Kidney 8-Lung 9-Heart 10-Liver 11-Colon.

The spleen is on the pad of the thumb; and the liver, heart, lungs and kidneys are on the pads of the index, middle, ring and little fingers respectively. The colon is on the radial border of the index finger from the tip to the web border of this finger; the small intestine is on the ulnar border of the little finger from the tip to the proximal end of this finger; the tip of little finger is Shending (vertex of kidney) and the distal palmar interphalangeal crease is called Shenwen (kidney crease); the proximal palmar interphalangeal creases of the index, middle, ring and little fingers are called Sihengwen (4 creases); the palmar metacarpophalangeal creases of 4 fingers are called Xiao-

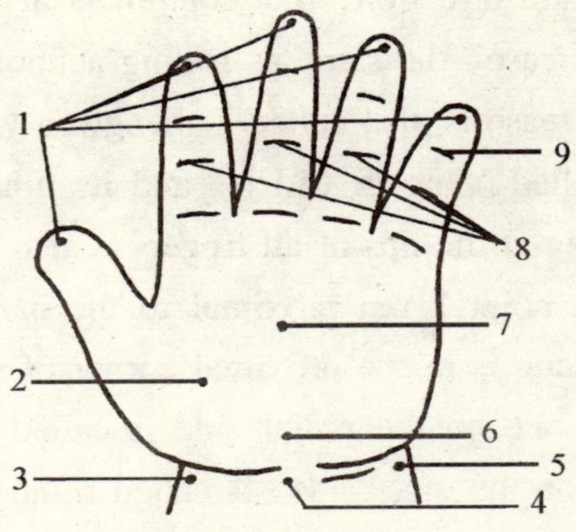

Fig. 6-3

1-Shiwang (Shixuan) 2-Banmen 3-Yangchi (LI 5) 4-Zongjin 5-Yinchi 6-Small Tianxin 7-Inner Laogong (PC 8) 8-Sihengwen (4 creases) 9-Shenwen

hengwen (small crease); the palmar crease proximal to the Xiaohengwen is called Zhang Xiaohengwen (small palmar crease); and the stomach is on the palmar side of metacarpophalangeal joint. In addition, the palmar surface of thenar prominence is called Banmen, the center of the palm is called Inner Laogong (PC 8) at a point between the tips of the middle and ring fingers when they are flexed to touch the palm; the Inner Bagua is a circle at the central part of the palm two-thirds of the distance between the center of the palm and proximal end of the middle finger as its radius; the Small Tianxin is in a depression between thenar and hypothenar prominences; the arc of Yunshui Rutu is drawn from proximal end of the little finger to proximal end of the thumb and the arc of Yuntu Rushui is drawn along the opposite direction; the Zongjin is at the midpoint of palmar carpal crease, the same as Daling acupoint (PC 7); the palmar carpal crease is also called Dahengwen (big crease), its radial end is called Yangchi (LI 5) and its ulnar end is called Yinchi; Shiwang at the tips of all fingers is also called Shixuan; Laolong is at a point 1 fen proximal to the nail of the middle finger; Duanzheng is at the proximal corner of nail of the middle finger, the one on the radial side is called left Duanzheng and the other, on the ulnar side, is called right Duanzheng; the dorsal creases of proximal interphalangeal joints of the 5 fingers are called Wuzhijie (5 interphalangeal creases); the points in the depressions beside the proximal end of the middle finger are called Ershanmen; Shangmen is in the depression between the proximal ends of the ring and little fingers; the Outer Laogong is on the dorsum of the hand and just opposite to the Inner Laogong; Weiling is in the interosseous space between the 2nd and 3rd metacarpal bones, and Jingning is in the interosseous space between the 4th and 5th metacarpal bones; the Outer Bagua is on the dorsum of the hand and opposite to the Inner Bagua; and Yiwofeng is at the midpoint of dorsal carpal crease.

For child health care massage, the kneading, pinching or pinching with grinding maneuvers may be applied at the tips of all fingers; kneading maneuver applied to the pads of all fingers; and the pushing or grinding with pushing maneuvers applied along radial or ulnar borders of the fingers. The local grinding and pushing maneuvers applied to the correspondent reflecting areas of internal organs are a toning technique; and the vertical pushing maneuver applied along fingers is a reducing technique. The vertical pushing maneuver proximally applied along colon and small intestine reflecting areas is a toning technique and the distally applied is a reducing technique. The pressing with kneading and pinching with grinding maneuvers are usually applied over reflecting areas; and the pinching and pushing maneuvers applied at acupoints.

The procedures for child health care massage are arranged as follows: To tone spleen and reduce stomach for adjusting digestive tract and to reduce heart and liver for adjusting function of lung and kidney; to digit-press, press and knead Banmen and Duanzheng, to transport water into earth and to motivate Bagua; to manage Hengwen (creases) and Zongjin for clearing heat and releasing stasis; and to manage Outer Laogong and points and reflecting areas called Men and Feng for expelling external pathogens; and to manage Tianxin, Laogong and carpal crease for improving the health of children and preventing disease. Other points and reflecting areas can also be selected for use according to necessity and under the guidance of the practitioner. The acupoints and reflecting areas at the distal end of the fingers, such as Shiwang, can be used for emergency treatment. The persistent application of health care massage once or twice a day may improve the health of children, prevent disease and promote the development of their intelligence. In addition, children should be trained to constantly use their hands, for example to pick up and hold things, clap their hands, and play with building blocks to improve their coordination of movement between hands and brain. Before and after massage, their hands should be soaked in warm water, and they should be trained apt to receive a warm-water soaking of hands and feet. It's a delicate job, and health care should be continuously carried on with hand massage adequately applied with the proper force to avoid injuring the child's tender hands.

2. Foot massage for child health care

The foot massage is also very important for children. The central part of the sole, heel and toes, especially the big toe, are the important places for applying massage, and the joints of the foot, especially the ankle and first metatarsophalangeal joint, are also very important.

The procedures for child foot massage are as follows:

1) Rubbing foot:

The rubbing maneuver may be quickly and gently applied with the whole ulnar border of palm, from the ankle joint over instep (including the medial and laterl borders of the foot) to toes; and then from the heel tendon over heel and sole to toes with a force heavier than that used for the instep. For rubbing the midline of the sole, the lateral border of hypothenar prominence may be used instead. The rubbing maneuver producing a pink color and a hot sensation all over the child's feet may promote their growth and development, clear heat in body, remove food stagnation, induce sweating, and expel pathogens from the body surface.

2) Pushing foot:

The pushing maneuver is forcefully applied from the midpoint of lateral border of the heel along the lateral and medial dorsoplantar boundary of the foot to the little and big toes respectively, and then the gentle rotating, digit-pressing and kneading maneuvers are applied to the little and big toes. The pushing maneuver is useful to clear heat, control convulsions, refresh the mind, open the sense organs, and enhance intelligence.

3) Digit-pressing and kneading joints:

The digit-pressing and kneading maneuvers are applied from the ankle joint through the 1st to the 5th metatarsophalangeal joints, and finally the gentle digit-pressing maneuver is applied to all interphalangeal joints. The manipulation should be gently and nimbly applied with a proper amplitude of movement. The digit-pressing and kneading manipulation can promote the development of the child's muscular and skeletal system, and the pinching and digit-pressing manipulation can be used to treat emergency cases of convulsions, but this must be quickly and accurately applied.

4) Grinding and pressing central part of sole:

The quick, gentle and nimble grinding and pressing maneuvers are applied over the central part and the part slightly anterior to the center of the sole for clearing heat, control vomiting, and promoting digestion in the spleen and stomach.

5) Gently pounding heel:

The ulnar borders of both fists are used to quickly and rhythmically pound the heels with a proper and even force for tranquilizing the mind, improving sleep, and controlling convulsions.

6) Rubbing foot:

The first manipulation is repeated as the closing step in this set of manipulations.

The feet should be soaked in warm water before applying the above manipulations, and after the foot bath, the warmth of the feet should be retained because an attack of cold to the feet may cause other diseases. The health care foot massage may be performed alone or combined with hand massage, and the frequency of manipulation may be increased. Young babies should not be forced to begin walking at a very young age because this may disturb the body's development and cause deformity of the bones and joints. Babies should be supported when walking so their legs do not carry all their body weight at the early stages of learning to walk.

Before the practitioner begins the child health care massage on hand and foot, he/she should wash his/her hands in warm water and have his/her nails cut short to avoid injury. People with hard skin, hard scars and scales on the skin, or other lesions on their hands should not use their hands to do this massage. The manipulation should be carefully applied without any violence to avoid injury. If this massage is done at home, it is best done by mothers, because sometimes men may injure the child by applying too much force.

Young children are very susceptible to attacks of pathogens because their body resistance is not yet fully strengthened. At the same time, the development of disease in children may be very rapid, and neglecting the seriousness of their illness may produce an incurable result. Therefore, young parents must not carelessly manage the disease of their children, and they should visit the pediatrician in time.

III. Hand and Foot Hygiene

The hand and foot massage and exercise include the care of the hand and foot themselves. The adequate use of the hand and foot in daily life, the correct selection of ordinary protective matrials such as cosmetic, gloves and shoes, and hygiene and sanitary care are also very important.

1. Hand hygiene

The hand is the most useful and skillful part of the body, built with complicated anatomical structures and capable of multiple functions. Two important problems must be considered because of the close contact of the hands with surrounding substances. The first is protection of the hand. In clinical practice, many patients with hand injuries must be treated by the surgeons, and many cases have functional impairment or even a lifelong disability. Therefore, particular care must be taken to protect the hands from injury. The second important problem is hand hygiene because the hands are always contacting surrounding substances, either clean or dirty. A large number of pathogens may be present in the fissures of nails and creases of the hands, and these may be brought into the mouth with food, possibly leading to disease. So care must be taken to prevent food-born diseases transmitted by hand. At the same time, diseases of the hand itself must be treated in time to guard against future trouble.

Hand washing is the best method to keep the hands clean. Sterilizing soap, ordinary soap, or a soap solution may be selected for people with different types of skin. The fissures, borders and grooves of the nails, and the fissures and creases of the fingers should be carefully washed to remove any hidden dirt. The nails are best trimmed after they are soaked in a warm soapy solution until they become soft. The nails should be neither cut too short nor grown too long, and the nail spine should be carefully cut away. The free edge of the nail should be cut into an arc curve and filed to form a smooth border.

Gloves are also very important for hand care. Protective gloves should be the right size for easy wear. Gloves for keeping hands clean should be made of compact cloth rather than netted material and should be worn after the hands have been washed. Gloves for preserving warmth should be the right size because the very loose gloves will not preserve warmth, and very tight gloves may interfere with blood circulation. Gloves are an important clothing accessory, and the correct selection and wearing of gloves is very useful in health care.

Cosmetic and skin care materials for the hand are also important. The quality of skin care materials is determined by their ability to moist, soften and nourish the skin, not by their fragrance or price. The skin care materials in an oil base are good for dry skin, and a water base is good for oily skin; and a diluted oil base is best for normal skin. The skin care materials should not be applied to hands with skin lesions, and after the skin lesions are healed the application of these materials must follow the advice of a dermatologist. In general, after the hands are washed and soaked in warm water for a while, the water on the hand is dried with a towel and a thin layer of glycerol is applied over the skin. Then the skin care materials may be applied. Many girls prefer to paint their nails with colored nail oil. After the hand and nails are washed clean, one or two layer of transparent nail oil or protective nail ointment should be applied first before applying colored nail oil. Nail oil of any kind should be evenly applied from the center of the nail to its periphery, and the oil should be changed frequently otherwise it may become harmful. People should learn something about cosmetology if they want to correctly use cosmetic and skin care materials.

2. Foot hygiene

Like the hand, the security and cleanliness of the foot is also essential for preventing foot diseases and improving general health. The feet should be soaked in warm water after walking or exercising for a long time each night before going to bed. The warmth should be maintained after the feet are soaked and washed. The method for properly cutting the toenails is similar to that for the fingernails. Diseases of the foot must be treated in time to avoid future complications.

Socks should be soft in texture, the proper size and comfortable to wear; and they should be changed every day. Tight socks are not suitable because they may pressure the foot. Shoe-pads should fit the shoes and be made of soft, elastic, and absorbent material. Selection of the proper shoes is particularly important. The size and shape should fit the foot, and be slightly larger than the foot for comfortable wearing and walking. The shoes should be made of material with good ventilation and low heels. The pressure on the sole of the foot should be even. Several models of shoes are harmful to the foot. For example, pointed shoes may produce a squeezing action and cause poor blood circulation, pain, or even deformity of the metatarsophalangeal joints and toes. Shoes with very high heels are very harmful to the development of adolescent girls, and may cause "high-heel syndrome" or even death. And heavy boots may inhibit walking movement of the body. If possible walking and running on bare feet is encouraged, because the ground can produce a healthy rubbing effect on the feet. Sneakers are also a good choice because their scientific design is beneficial.

In brief, the correct selection of foot wear is very important in the care of the foot; and pleasant and comfortable walking is enjoyable and good exercise.

IV. Hand and Foot Massage Helpful for Maintaining Health and Prolonging Life

After reading this book, you may have some understanding of the acupoints and reflecting areas, massage, diagnosis, and care of the hand and foot. The authors hope the knowledge obtained from this book and strengthened by your own practice may help to improve your health and the health of others, and that eventually hand and foot massage may become a good friend.

As an important component of the traditional Chinese medical treasury, hand and foot massage was created in the course of the Chinese people's intelligent and productive struggle against disease. It is a treasury belonged to the people, and anyone has the right to study and develop it, as well as to enjoy the benefits of primary health care. It may be considered a part of the foundation stone for building the hall of people's health.

Finally, in learning hand and foot massage, the general principles, including studying assiduously and with perseverence, advancing step by step, and improving skills through practice should be followed. In addition to this book, the reader is invited and encouraged to read other books and make every effort to practise and develop his skills.

We hope hand and foot massage will be helpfuf for maintaining health and prolonging life.

图书在版编目（CIP）数据

中国传统手足按摩法：英文/吴更伟，郝东方著.
一北京：外文出版社，2001
ISBN 7-119-01945-7
I. 中… Ⅱ. ①吴… ②郝… Ⅲ. ①手-按摩疗法（中医）-英文
② 足-按摩疗法（中医）-英文 Ⅳ. R 244 .1
中国版本图书馆 CIP 数据核字（97）第 10123 号

责任编辑　　胡开敏
英文编辑　　李含春
封面设计　　陈　军
插图绘制　　程星涛
印刷监制　　冯　浩

外文出版社网址：
http://www.flp.com.cn
外文出版社电子信箱：
info@flp.com.cn
sales@flp.com.cn

中国传统手足按摩法

吴更伟　郝东方　著
*

©外文出版社
外文出版社出版
（中国北京百万庄大街 24 号）
邮政编码　100037
北京蓝空印刷厂印刷
中国国际图书贸易总公司发行
（中国北京车公庄西路 35 号）
北京邮政信箱第 399 号　邮政编码　100044
2001 年（大 32 开）第 1 版
2001 年第 1 版第 1 次印刷
（英）
ISBN 7-119-01945-7/R.143（外）
05000（平）
14-E-3135 P